# VIEW FROM THE DECK

Recollections of the 10th Annual Voyage

of the CGS C.D. Howe, 1959

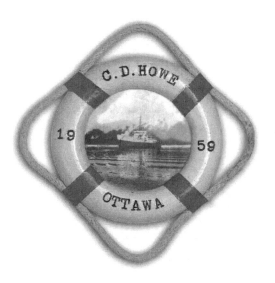

*This souvenir was purchased by the author while on board the
CGS* C.D. Howe *in 1959. The life preserver ring was handcrafted from
wood by the ship's carpenter. The braided rope around the ring shows signs
of being in storage as well as many years of handling. The picture inside
the ring was taken by the carpenter while the* Howe *rode at anchor in the
Arctic. It was recently refurbished, and the image was enhanced
by the late Ralph Buttrum of Perth, Ontario.*

# View from the Deck

Recollections of
the 10th Annual Voyage
of the CGS C.D. Howe, 1959

## Murray Ault

Published by Murray Ault

ISBN 978-0-9949220-0-7 (pbk.)
ISBN 978-0-9949220-1-4 (epub)
ISBN 978-0-9949220-2-1 (mobi)

Copyright © Murray Ault 2014

Cover art, design: Magdalene Carson / New Leaf Publication Design

Printed and bound in Canada

Cataloguing in Publication data available at Library and Archives Canada

*This book is dedicated to all who share a passion of the North, as well as to those who have visited, lived and worked, and explored the mysteries and grandeur of Canada's northern realm, and who have established lasting friendships with our northern neighbours. In your heart of hearts, you know you have an enduring affinity to the many and varied aspects of this part of Canada. May your memories serve to encourage others to share your passion. The record of your travels and experiences will serve as a legacy for all who may follow in your footsteps.*

*IN MEMORY OF*

*My mother, father, and sister Carolyn (Susie).*

*William (Bill) Watters (1941–63), seaman,*
*CGS d'Iberville 1959*

*Following our Arctic adventures, Bill and I spent the summer of 1960 on a bicycle tour of Europe, travelling as far east as Ankara, Turkey, where we spent two weeks with Bill's parents. His dad was a professor at the American University in Ankara under the auspices of the UN. Bill's untimely and tragic death occurred in December 1963. He is greatly missed by his family and many friends.*

*Michael (Mike) Harris (1939–2012), seaman,*
*CGS N.B. McLean 1959*

*Upon successful completion of his secondary school education, Mike entered the retail business. We would often pick up conversations from where we had left off during our last visit. Mike had a successful career in sales with the E.R. Fisher Company in Ottawa.*

*Ruth McLeese, MD (1932–2013), medical officer,*
*CGS C.D. Howe 1959*

*Ruth and I shared a three-month journey on the Eastern Arctic Patrol aboard the CGS C.D. Howe in 1959. On completion of her medical studies, her first assignment was as a medical officer on the Howe. Over the past three years while writing this book, I considered myself fortunate to renew my acquaintance with Dr. McLeese. In my letters to her, I attached chapters, hoping that her comments would help me add some colour to the material. Oftentimes, she did comment, but stated that many of her recollections were fuzzy.*

*As I was approaching completion of the book, I looked forward to having a few words of wisdom from Ruth. That was not to be, and I was devastated to discover that Ruth had passed away. While her last note to me expressed her sadness with the passing of her dog Charlie, her beloved and faithful companion, there was no indication that her health was failing.*

*Ruth's life was a celebration unto itself. She gave of herself for the benefit of others, and I was saddened by this loss. She was a talented lady who had many interesting facets, as exhibited by an excerpt from CARP magazine she once included in a letter. It was a picture of her beside her aircraft. That image brought back a recollection of her enjoying helicopter rides that summer of 1959, as she took her skills and compassion to the Inuit people.*

# Table of Contents

|  | Acknowledgements | ix |
|  | Apologia | xiii |
|  | Preface | xv |
| Chapter One | Homecoming | 1 |
| Two | Beginnings | 6 |
| Three | Northward Bound | 23 |
| Four | In the Straits, Part I: Hudson Strait | 35 |
| Five | In the Straits, Part II: Hudson Strait Again | 51 |
| Six | The Port of Churchill, Hudson Bay | 66 |
| Seven | On to the Arctic Circle | 72 |
| Eight | Crossing the Arctic Circle, Davis Strait | 81 |
| Nine | Resolute Bay, Cornwallis Island, Lancaster Sound | 90 |
| Ten | Grise Fiord, Ellesmere Island, Jones Sound | 107 |
| Eleven | Pond Inlet, Baffin Island | 114 |
| Twelve | Cape Christian to Cape Dyer, Baffin Island, Davis Strait | 120 |
| Thirteen | Pangnirtung, Baffin Island, Cumberland Sound | 123 |
| Fourteen | Frobisher Bay, Baffin Island | 128 |
| Fifteen | Homeward Bound | 133 |
|  | Afterword | 138 |
| Appendix A | Interview with Liz Delaute Simms and Suzanne Delaute Allan | 139 |
| Appendix B | The Eastern Arctic Patrol | 150 |
| Appendix C | Statistical Information | 154 |
| Appendix D | Manifest 1959 (unofficial) | 157 |
|  | Bibliography | 160 |
|  | About the Author | 162 |

# Acknowledgements

Many have assisted in writing this book. While a book is recognized as the work of mbedthe author, the final product could never come to be without the behind-the-scenes efforts of those who have given their time and knowledge to assist the author. Such has been my case. Below is a small "thank you" to the many who have contributed in their own way. Their assistance is appreciated by the author.

I extend heartfelt thanks to my wife Judie. She has been by my side throughout the long process of writing and editing. She has helped by going to libraries for research materials, checking spelling and punctuation, and has endured the many hours of my being before the computer. Her assistance and forbearance have been stellar. I am most appreciative of her knowledge of words and skills as a wordsmith.

I am indebted to Dr. Ruth McLeese, of Hampton, New Brunswick, who served as medical officer on board the *C.D. Howe* in 1959. She joined the Eastern Arctic Patrol upon graduation from medical school at Dalhousie University in Halifax. I was fortunate to link up with Dr. Ruth through the internet and Canada Post, and we corresponded as she took time away from her famous garlic garden. She also shared several of her personal photos taken during the patrol, many of which capture the images of those who came aboard the ship for their medicals. These are timeless pictures that tell a story all their own. Other images, specifically those taken from the cockpit of the helicopter, are invaluable. I cherish them all. They add colour to the story.

Thank you also to Helen Gamble of Perth, Ontario. I met Helen through our mutual affiliation in a service club, where I discovered she enjoyed writing books, articles, and short stories. When I mentioned my idea of writing a book, she offered to help me get up and running. It was through her efforts that I got going on the "write" path.

During the initial writing stages, I contacted the Reference Section of the Library and Archives of Canada (LAC) for documents related to the Eastern Arctic Patrol. Claire Banton replied with a list of documents related to the Eastern Arctic Patrol 1945–60, and through interlibrary loan, I was able to review the material at my leisure. For this, I thank Claire. Her assistance helped me get on the right track.

I would be remiss if I did not thank the staff at the Clarington Public Library in Newcastle and Bowmanville, in particular, librarians Annette Helmecke-Moore and Soi Mui Chau. Their assistance was invaluable as I stumbled along in my research. They kept encouraging me with each resource I requested.

For Chapter 14, "Frobisher Bay, Baffin Island," I decided to track down Liz Delaute, whom I was pleased to discover lived in Ottawa. The result of this fortunate reconnection appears in Appendix A. Both Liz Delaute Simms and her sister Suzanne Delaute Allan shared their recollections of living in Frobisher Bay with their parents during 1959. Liz also sent me pictures of the site, some of which I have included. Their contribution has enhanced my knowledge and understanding of living in the North. Who would believe a brief encounter on the *C.D. Howe* more than fifty years ago would bring forth a wider scope to this adventure.

A number of years ago, I was fortunate to catch an interview on the CBC radio program, "Morningside," on the relocation of Eskimo families from Port Harrison (Quebec) to Craig Harbour, Ellesmere Island. The salient point was the relocation carried out by the CGS *C.D. Howe* in 1953. Host Peter Gzowski was interviewing Professor Shelagh Grant, history professor at Trent University. Dr. Grant wrote an article, "A Case of Compound Error: The Inuit Resettlement Project 1953, and the Government Response, 1990," which was published in *Northern Perspectives*, Vol. 19, No. 1 (Spring 1991). I have excerpted portions of this article elsewhere in this book. Dr. Grant inspired me to complete my book project, and I extend my thanks to Dr. Grant for her encouragement.

I would also like to add my thanks to the following for their time and care in helping this book come to fruition.

Elizabeth Hawkins, Vancouver, retired from Library and Archives Canada after an interesting career. She researched the last known whereabouts of the *C.D. Howe* at the Maritime Museum in Vancouver. Our emails were a chance to delve into some personal connections we shared in Ottawa, which were illuminating to say the least. Thank you, Elizabeth, for adding insight and clearing up misconceptions.

Charles Maginley, co-author with Bernard Collin of *The Ships of Canada's Marine Services*. I found this book helpful on several occasions, as there were several ships serving in the North at the time the *Howe* was on patrol. To see images of the *Howe* as she commenced her journey from Montreal brought back fond recollections. Charles, I thank you as well for responding to my inquiries.

On a closing note, I am indebted to many who have encouraged me to develop and complete this project. You have helped to bring glimpses of our Arctic regions and individuals for others to discover and enjoy.

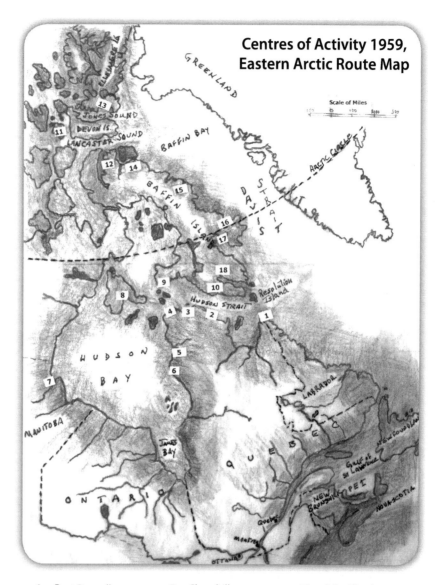

**Centres of Activity 1959, Eastern Arctic Route Map**

Scale of Miles

| | | |
|---|---|---|
| 1. Port Burwell | 7. Churchill | 13. Grise Fiord |
| 2. Wakeham Bay | 8. Coral Harbour | 14. Pond Inlet |
| 3. Sugluk | 9. Cape Dorset | 15. Clyde River |
| 4. Ivujivik | 10. Lake Harbour | 16. Padloping Island |
| 5. Povungnituk | 11. Resolute Bay | 17. Pangnirtung |
| 6. Port Harrison | 12. Arctic Bay | 18. Frobisher Bay |

(Author's collection)

# Apologia

The People of the Eastern Arctic inhabit a vast territory. Originally, they lived in small settlements near their sources of food. One may characterize these people as courageous and tenacious, but never as foolhardy. Their skills to carve out a livelihood under harsh living conditions stand as a testament to their ingenuity. Their stories, which comprise their history, objets d'art, paintings, and songs reflect the salient features of living in an inhospitable environment.

At the time of events in this book, these people were referred to in English as Eskimos. Today, they are respectfully referred to as Inuit. Similarly, place names have been changed to the accepted Inuit names. For example, Frobisher Bay is today known as Iqaluit, while others include Cape Dorset (Kinngait), Lake Harbour (Kimmirut), and Port Harrison (Inukjuak).

Thus, this author apologizes for using the word Eskimo in reference to the Inuit people and retaining English placenames in lieu of the correct Inuit names. This practice was not, nor ever considered to be a negative connotation towards these people whose very life, history, and traditions have brought character and history to the Canadian North.

# Preface

There I was at eighteen years of age, six weeks from sitting the dreaded final provincial exams, anticipating completing secondary school, and looking forward to a unique summer job. My heart was set on working as a cabin boy on board the CGS *C.D. Howe*. It promised to be a singular experience to work and travel in the far northern regions of Canada. At this stage of my young life, the Arctic was but a vague concept gleaned from geography studies and newspaper articles.

Chuck Everett, a school chum, had worked as a cabin steward the previous summer on the *Howe*. At every opportunity, I questioned him about his experiences. His answers only led to even more questions. I was intrigued.

Each day after sending in my application, I hurried home from school and rifled through the mail hoping there would be a letter of acceptance from the Department of Transport. Finally, around the middle of May 1959, there arrived a large brown envelope with the Department of Transport printed in the upper left-hand corner. I quickly tore open the envelope. To my delight, it was my hoped-for good news. "You have been selected as a Cabin Steward," it said, "to serve on board the Canadian Government Ship *C.D. Howe*." I was overjoyed.

Further on, I read that I was to report for duty at the Port of Montreal, Shed 62, on June 25, 1959, at 0630 hours, along with other instructions pertaining to being properly prepared for this trip. So much to do with so little time in which to do it.

More than half a century has passed since my time as member of the crew on the tenth annual voyage of the CGS *C.D. Howe*. I kept a diary that summer, essentially a travelogue of sorts, "a view from the deck," in which the adventures of the *Howe* and those who sailed with her were recorded. This was the first Canadian-built ship designed specifically to provide medical and dental services to the inhabitants of the Eastern Arctic.

That diary, as well as letters sent home to my parents, formed the basis for this book. Although the voyage was brief—only three months—it was a watershed event in both my life and that of the North.

For many years, expeditions into the Canadian North may be characterized as intermittent forays, most notably voyages led by Captain Joseph E. Bernier in the early years of the twentieth century. Others included whalers originating from faraway ports and explorers seeking the elusive Northwest Passage.

On July 1, 1925, Captain Bernier departed Quebec City at the helm of the *Arctic* with twenty-six officers and crew. Eskimo Nokudlah, who had been sentenced to ten years of imprisonment for murder, was being returned to Pond Inlet on early parole. Diagnosed with tuberculosis, he was a patient of Dr. Leslie D. Livingstone, who was also on board along with several RCMP officers.

Dudley Copeland, in his book, *Livingstone of the Arctic*, recounts the experiences of Dr. Livingstone and his demonstrated concern for the health and well-being of the Eskimos. This expedition coincided with the time that the Canadian government started taking an interest in the well-being of the dwellers of this region.

Reports back to Ottawa indicated that the Eskimos lived an individual and isolated life. One may wonder how they survived in such an inhospitable and cruel environment. But live they did. Their history, culture, and lifestyle have been passed down through the generations through their art, sculpture, song, and dance, the genesis of which can be found in the stories told in the dim, flickering light of the seal oil lamps in the confines of cozy igloos. Theirs was a way of life that today has become largely the stuff of history books.

After the Second World War, annual voyages by government ships into this remote region of Canada opened up contact with the outside world. The expansion of communication links may be seen with the development of federal government services, the growth of the number of Hudson's Bay outlets, the addition of RCMP detachments, and the establishment of churches in the many scattered communities. In addition, the settlements of Frobisher Bay and Resolute Bay boasted weather stations, military bases, and extensive airport facilities. These and many other changes impacted the Eskimos' way of life.

One could foresee that, in the not too distant future, great change—both positive and negative—was coming for the Eskimos.

This voyage and my contact with them certainly changed my life.

# Chapter One

# Homecoming

The CGS *C.D. Howe* had been my home away from home since the 25th of June. Exactly three months had passed, and this was my last day on board. We had been ninety-three days at sea. Days filled with amazing sights, adventures, and an untold number of memorable moments.

There had been an atmosphere of anxious anticipation among all aboard for the past few days. A combination of expectation of the conclusion of the voyage and arriving home, referred to as "channel fever." I had packed my duffel bag many times over during the past several days, leaving out only a few essential items that I could stuff in at a moment's notice. I had adopted this ritual so as, hopefully, to speed the passage of time and close the distance to our final destination.

On this special bright, sunny day, the ship sailed under a full head of steam towards Quebec City. Travelling up the St. Lawrence, I watched the picturesque scenery from the Promenade Deck. It is no wonder that people from all over the world come to visit this area, as it is beautiful—a breathtaking panorama of trees, mountains, and rugged coastline. Mother Nature's paint brush had dressed the trees in vibrant orange, red, and yellow, leaving a few hints of green still to peek through.

With our chores completed, we joined the farewell party already in progress in the lounge, where the conversation was light and jovial. Each had a story to tell, and the lounge rang with chatter and laughter as we made short work of the tasty snacks, dessert goodies, and beverages on offer. The conversations took our minds off the pending sadness of our eventual goodbyes. I myself had made several friends among the ship's officers, the medical staff, the hydrographic engineers, and the seamen, as well as with the postmaster, the night steward, and the ship's carpenter. Everybody was in a happy mood.

Within a few hours, the *Howe* would be moored alongside the quay in Quebec City, her engines shut down, and the *Howe*'s tenth annual voyage would be over. Passengers and crew would disperse to the far corners of Canada, home at last.

Although obviously busy with a few last-minute jobs, the chief steward approached me to say that the captain wished to see me in his cabin. This was unusual. Usually it was the duty of the chief steward to give us our orders or admonish us for some task overlooked. What could he want, especially as we were nearing the conclusion of the voyage? Dreadful thoughts passed swiftly through my mind. What on earth had I done? I thought back to my first day on ship when I met him over the issue of the "lost papers." I stood anxiously outside the open door of the captain's cabin.

First Mate Pelletier spoke up, "Please come in."

I was still dressed in my steward's jacket, and if I had a cap, I would have held it my hands as I humbly entered the cabin.

"As you know," the captain began, "in a few hours we will be alongside at Quebec. The final hours of your service on board will be ending soon, and there is the small detail of signing off on the ship's register. Please sit here and sign this." He placed a postcard-sized document on the table.

I sat in the offered chair, read the document, and, when presented with a pen, signed my name on the black line. The captain then gave me the completed "Certificate of Discharge" and shook my hand. That was it! I stood up, expressed my thanks, and left the cabin.

Outside the cabin, I stopped and took a closer look at the certificate. I noted that my character for conduct and ability to serve in any capacity was rated VG. I was most pleased that in the eyes of the captain I had served well and was rated as "very good."

I still had to finish a few additional chores, returning the mops, brooms, sponges and pails, polishing clothes and brass cleaner, rags, cleansers, and my steward's jacket to their respective closets. I was glad to shed these trappings of the job and was now looking forward to registering for school and returning to my studies.

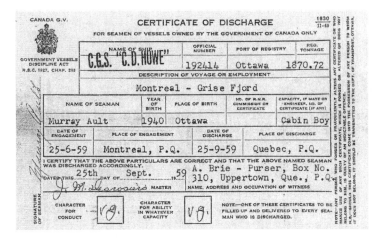

*Certificate of Discharge. Author's collection.*

In the early afternoon, the historic city of Quebec came into view. I went out onto the Promenade Deck to get a better look. I recognized the topmost spires and the familiar structure of the famed Château Frontenac. As we approached the quay, I could see La Terrace where we spent a warm June evening before we sailed, strolling, talking about the forthcoming voyage, and taking in all the delightful images.

I never tired of watching the process involved in mooring the ship. I stationed myself in the bow area, previously off limits, to observe the seamen as they grabbed the heavy lines for securing the ship to the quay. As I leaned against the side of the ship, my mind flashed back to that day in Churchill, the last time we had been alongside a quay, when we cast off knowing full well the next time we would be at a mooring would be at Quebec. That was many weeks ago, many miles of sea travelled, and many intriguing and memorable experiences.

Off the starboard bow, families and friends were standing and waving as the ship inched its way slowly alongside the quay. Several members of the medical staff joined me, and we scanned the crowd in hopes of seeing familiar faces. The scene was reminiscent of arrivals at a settlement in the Far North.

I searched the crowd carefully trying to find my family, but as much as I wished to see them, they were nowhere to be seen. Several dark thoughts rushed through my mind. Had my parents received my letters informing them of the date and approximate time of our expected arrival at Quebec? Were my hopes for a joyful reunion to be dashed? Was this another example of my father's habit of arriving late? Perhaps the wireless officer had received a radiogram from Ottawa stating that my parents were not able to come to pick me up and I was to seek alternative transportation home? I feared that I would not experience a proper welcome.

Once the ship was secured to the quay and the gangplank was lowered, many of those on board disembarked to greet their families. It was a heartwarming sight watching many of my friends and crew mates mingling in a state of happiness and relief that the voyage had ended safely.

Then, off in the distance, I recognized the family car as it made its way down to the quay and all my dark thoughts quickly dissipated. With misty eyes, I threaded my way through the boisterous crowd to meet my family. We exchanged hugs many times over amongst a flood of questions from my parents and siblings. At the same time, I wanted to introduce them to the friends I had made on the voyage. It was a time of confusion, trying to do too many things at once. I suggested we go on board for a tour in hopes their many questions would be answered.

"What is that strange feeling?" my ten-year-old sister, Christie, asked. "The ship seems to be rolling from side to side."

"Is this normal, rocking back and forth? Is there any danger?" asked my mother with a hint of concern in her voice.

"I don't feel any rocking," I replied. "I am sure this is normal with so many people on board." I hoped this would assuage Mum's fears. Several months ago during a bout of seasickness, the quartermaster had said that I would get my sea legs. Now I realized what he had meant.

The several levels of decks, the passageways, the solid steel bulkheads, the steep, narrow stairs of the companionways, and the hand rails—all were second nature to me. After three months of living on board, I could navigate the interior of the ship with ease. On the other hand, my mother, unfamiliar with these features of the ship, urged me not to go too fast. As tour director, I was hurrying from one part of the ship to another, anxious that they got to see as much of the ship as possible. My siblings also asked me to slow down. This was a whole new experience for them.

We descended to the lowest deck so that I could show them the living quarters I had shared with three other cabin mates. We had called our cabin the "Executive Suite," even though it was neither executive, nor was it a suite.

"This was where you lived for the past three months!" cried my mother. "How could you live in this?" Dad and my siblings quietly cast their eyes around the cabin, taking in all the little things we had done to spruce up our home. The expressions on their faces switched quickly from wonder to distaste.

Suddenly, it became dead quiet. Everyone had a quizzical look on their faces.

"What happened?" asked my brother and father almost simultaneously. "How come it is so quiet down here now? When we first came down there was a constant, loud cranking noise."

"That noise you heard was coming from the engine room," I replied. "It was a constant noise while we were under way at sea. I guess the captain gave the order, 'Finished with all engines.'" This was another sign that we were home to stay.

"Let's go and see another part of the ship," stated my father, anxious to leave my cramped quarters. I guess the reality was much different than what I had described in my many letters home.

We continued our tour through the ship: the galleys, where meals were prepared; the mess areas for the seamen; the dining salon with the panorama windows; the Boat Deck and safety equipment; and the medical suite with operating rooms and the X-ray suite. We moved quickly, as it would soon be time to leave the ship. We gathered my duffel bag and other personal belongings. The only thing left to do was say final goodbyes to my sailing friends.

I recall my feelings at the end of this voyage. Although it had been a summer job that had far exceeded any other possibility, it was good to be home and in familiar surroundings. I looked forward to home-cooked meals, time with family and friends, as well as sleeping in my own, comfortable bed.

I was also eager to share with friends the wonders of the North and my experiences on board the CGS *C.D. Howe*, both good and not so good.

And now I have a chance to share those memories again.

# Chapter Two

# Beginnings

I first heard about the possibility of working on board the *C.D. Howe* from Chuck Everett, a school chum who had been hired as a cabin steward for the summer of 1958. After several conversations that left me with more questions than answers, I decided to take the plunge and submit my application to the Department of Transport. I crossed my fingers that I would be chosen.

My elation at being accepted as a cabin steward quickly turned to mild panic when I realized that I only had a few short weeks to get ready and there was much to be done. In addition to my letter of acceptance, I found documents that needed signing, lists of clothing and gear that I would need suited for the rigours of the North, and an itinerary of the *Howe*'s ports of call. I quickly realized the special nature of this three-month journey.

The clothing list stipulated that I have a duffel bag for clothing and accessories. I used my father's—a canvas tube with brass grommets through which a rope was threaded, suitable for closing and securing the bag. He had used it while overseas during the war. Although it was summer, I packed warm clothing; I had no idea how cold the weather would be.

The list also stated that I was to have two pairs of navy, woollen, bell-bottomed trousers. Assuming that these heavy items would take valuable space in my bag and be difficult to clean, I checked with Chuck, who said these trousers were not a necessity. He had packed only one pair and never wore them. This news resulted in great sighs of relief from me and my parents.

Other instructions focused on the realities of living on a ship for three months. In fact, it was clearly stated that on-board storage facilities were limited, so personal items had to be kept to a minimum. After packing writing materials and a few other items I considered necessities, I considered myself as ready as I ever would be for my forthcoming adventure.

Lastly, the letter stated the date and time for reporting to the ship at the Port of Montreal.

However, a nagging worry wriggled in the back of my mind. What had I so willingly agreed to undertake? While I knew I would be gone for three months, it had not yet occurred to me that I would be out of touch. There was no such thing as daily news broadcasts or newspapers where I was going. In fact, it was not until we were well into the voyage did I realize how isolated we were. I was also of a mind, somewhat naively, that when I returned everything would be the same. It was as if I was going on a short vacation.

At 4 a.m. on June 25, my father drove me to Dr. W.T. Kendall's home. The early hour did nothing for my father's mood.

The Kendalls had agreed to drive me and their son Bill, who was also joining the *Howe* as a cabin steward, to Montreal. This was my first meeting with Bill. He was about my height, build, and age, and during the drive to Montreal, we discovered that we had many things in common. We hit it off right from the start, which was good, as we were destined to spend the next three months in close confines together.

Ottawa, at that early hour, was akin to a mausoleum. It was so quiet, one could roll a bowling ball down Sparks Street and hit nothing until it came to a stop at the foot of the War Memorial. Dr. Kendall sped through the city above the stated limits, gliding through stoplights. This was a new experience for me. Presumably any police car who spotted us would think he was heading to a medical emergency, due to the "MD" on his licence plates.

Sitting in the back seat of the Kendalls' car, I tried to take in the unfamiliar sights of a brightly lit but sleeping city. All too soon, however, we crossed the city limits into the dark countryside. Our conversation ceased. Occasionally, I could see lights marking farms and villages as we drove east along Highway 17, but the only sound was the noise of the tires as the miles ticked by. The stillness opened up a time of reflection. I had left home to start a new adventure not quite alone, but alone just the same.

When we arrived at the Port of Montreal a couple of hours later, it, too, was quiet. After coming to a stop at Shed 62, we could see the *Howe* moored alongside the quay, but no people. We unloaded our belongings from the car and stood there silently. I took a quick look around trying to absorb all the unfamiliar sights.

Dr. Kendall broke the silence. "I must return to Ottawa," he said. "I have appointments this morning." Dr. and Mrs. Kendall then wished us, "Bon voyage," and I thanked them for their kindness in driving me to the ship. Reluctantly, we bade each other farewell.

What had I got myself into? It was early morning, and we were standing all alone on a dirty quay, waiting. I felt abandoned. Where were the scores of rugged longshoremen and stevedores, carrying gaff-like implements as they set forth to tackle the next piece of cargo? Where was the hustle and bustle that I expected would be a constant on the docks of Montreal? Everything was grey—the sky, the harbour, and the buildings—which only added to the unwelcoming atmosphere. Shed 62 had few distinguishing features. It was an empty, three-sided wooden structure with a slanted roof that looked as if it was thrown up in a hurry and could come down just as fast. The *Howe* had white bulwarks and upper works, a black hull, and buff masts and funnel. The whole scene looked like a black-and-white photo. Was this an omen for the voyage?

It was 6:30. We were on time, according to our instructions, yet there was no one to meet us.

Bill and I stood chatting on the quay, taking the opportunity to get to know each other, but at the same time puzzled as to what to do next. Eventually, a ship's officer approached us. "Are you the men who have come to join the ship?" he asked.

"Yes," we replied.

"Welcome aboard and follow me."

Relieved, we gathered up our duffel bags and followed the officer up the gangplank and onto the deck of the CGS *C.D. Howe*, our home away from home for the next three months. I was a little disappointed that we were not piped aboard by the bosun, as was the accepted custom in my eyes. We just slipped on board without fanfare.

We were taken to a cabin on the Promenade Deck and instructed to remain there, as someone would come and get us squared away. The cabin appeared to be quite comfortable. It was suitably appointed with a bunk bed and curtains, storage lockers, a porthole decorated with government-issued curtains, magazine racks alongside each bunk for books and magazines, and a water closet (bathroom with a sink and toilet). It was modest but suitable as shipboard accommodation, and we hoped this would be our assigned quarters.

I wanted to get settled immediately, so that I could establish my own space and know where I was going to put my head that night. I also wanted a tour of the ship. It seemed so big. But there would be no such luck in that department. It appeared that any exploration would have to be done during assigned tasks or after hours. I was sure that, left to my own, it might take weeks to become acclimatized to these new surroundings. In due course, however, an officer approached us and requested that we come to the captain's cabin where we would sign the ship's register and thus become loyal members of Her Majesty's ship in the service of the Canadian government.

In comparison to the cabin we had been shown, the captain's cabin looked homey. Called a day cabin, it was larger than others and was furnished with a desk/table and a few chairs. There were three portholes with attractive curtains. Through a door, there was a smaller room, which contained a bed, shelves, and closet, and another room with a toilet, sink, and shower.

The captain was slim with aquiline features and appeared to be over six feet tall; a scowl marked his sour face. He was dressed in what may be described as a working outfit; signing up the cabin boys obviously didn't merit wearing his dress uniform. Undoubtedly, he was burdened by a never-ending to-do list in preparation for our three-month journey into the North, all probably more important than this administrative task.

I must say I was shaking in my shoes when I was introduced to him. I had expected him to be happy to have us aboard. He welcomed me aboard in French and a smattering of English; a bilingual officer explained the procedure for signing and taking the oath in English. This was important legal business. We swore on the Bible to serve with diligence, honesty, and at all times to obey the captain's orders. This was the first time in my life I had to make such a solemn oath, and I was firmly bound to do my duty as witnessed by those present and by God.

Then the captain requested our official papers—notification from the Department of Transport that stated who we were and that we had been authorized to join the ship. Crestfallen, I realized that I had left my papers at home in Ottawa. To the best of my recollection, I was not aware that I had to present these papers upon joining the ship. I had assumed, incorrectly, that the Department of Transport would formally contact the ship and provide all the necessary information and documentation.

I had no problem interpreting the dismay and consternation on the captain's face, as an ugly thought flashed through my mind. Would I be ordered to leave the ship? If so, how would I get back to Ottawa? After some discussion with his officers in French, of which I was able to understand a small bit, it was agreed to accept me aboard as a cabin steward. I was relieved. My worst fear of being left quayside would not be realized.

The whole experience left me shaken. He looked at me in contempt, and dread flowed through my veins causing a cold shiver to run down my back.

After the signing-in ceremony, I sought to find a quick and easy solution to my papers problem. I returned to the cabin where I had dumped my belongings and decided, as it was still early, to phone my father long distance and explain the situation. I then jumped ship (in contravention of the ship's regulations I had just signed and sworn an oath to uphold) and ran in search of the nearest phone booth. Fortunately, there was one in Shed 62. I dialled my father's office. His secretary answered and without hesitation connected me.

I quickly explained the problem and the urgency to forward the necessary papers to me. I also tried to emphasize the fact that the captain was not at all pleased. I was aware that this incident could impact negatively on me for the next three months. My father stated that he would do his best. I thanked him and returned to the ship. No one confronted me or queried me as to my brief absence from the ship. Perhaps the whole matter could be resolved in a short period of time with little added fuss.

Shortly thereafter, the cabin stewards—four of us English boys—were addressed by Chief Steward Moreau. Dressed in his officer's uniform and standing a little over five-and-a-half feet tall, the chief was our boss. Despite his diminutive stature, his stern countenance and commanding pose left no doubt as to who was in charge.

The chief listed the daily tasks we were expected to perform, and informed us of our hours of work, as well as several housekeeping rules and regulations. All seemed quite straightforward. We learned the location of mops, brooms, and other cleaning paraphernalia, as well as the location of fresh linen and extra blankets. Then, we were fitted with our working apparel: a neat white jacket with buttons up the front and pockets on either side, which we were required to wear at all times while on duty. Thus, to all, our shipboard status was clearly identified. It was evident we were to be of service to the passengers and officers on the ship. Surely, this was *de rigueur* on all Her Majesty's ships.

My first job was to wash and wax the stairway from the Bridge Deck to the Boat Deck. I gathered up a pail, rags, scrub brushes, cleaning solutions, and wax, and proceeded to follow the chief steward to the prescribed location. I realized this stairway led from the door of the captain's cabin to the Bridge Deck, and it was quite clear that the captain and other officers made frequent use of these stairs. Was this a test of my cleaning skills? I immediately thought that should the captain appear, I would be directly under his eyes. Any missteps and my goose would be cooked.

The stairway was very steep with linoleum on the treads and a ribbed aluminium edge along the fore-edge of each step. It was dirty. The grime had been well worn into the ribbing of the steps. This was a task requiring lots of hot, soapy water and elbow grease, and I suspected this stairway had not been cleaned since the last time the ship was in service. I got down to work.

I feared I would suffer another black mark if the completed job was less than perfect. My mind conjured up different kinds of punishment, all painful. This was the captain's access to the

Bridge. How often did he use these stairs each day? I was not going to shirk my duty now.

I decided to start at the top of the stairs, from where I had full view of the chart room, the wireless/radio equipment, and the main workings of the Bridge. I was fascinated by the layout of the Bridge and the array of electronic equipment that I could see from the top step. I knew I would never be invited to visit the Bridge and have the grand tour, so I stopped dreaming of the impossible and bent to my immediate task. I had not progressed very far when I overheard the voice of the wireless operator responding to an incoming message. I listened, curious as to the contents of the message, but could not make out even the gist of it, so I got on with my job. I decided that I would not start the next step until the step I was cleaning was pristine.

Then I heard a summons for me to report to the captain's cabin. What misdemeanour had I committed? Did he know about my off-ship foray to place a phone call home?

"Ottawa has contacted the ship by wireless and confirmed your authorized presence on the ship," the captain scowled. I was sure that the fact a cabin boy had influence in Ottawa to resolve the issue of his missing papers through a wireless message was the source of his displeasure. I was surely a marked man, now. I would be on the captain's radar for the duration of the voyage.

Regardless, my father had come through, and I was happy that all was in order. I assumed that the case of the missing papers had been put to rest.

I returned to washing the stairs, as I was convinced the captain would pay special attention to their cleanliness. Whether or not my diligence made a favourable impression on him, I do not know. I did know, however, that I would hear of any displeasure through the chief steward.

Fortunately, he was pleased with my work. "You have done a fine job," he reported upon inspection. "After lunch, we will go to the dining salon to wash and wax the floor there. Now go to lunch and report back at one o'clock."

"Where is lunch being served?" I asked.

"The Stewards' Mess. Just follow some of the seamen and you will find it," he replied offhandedly.

I made my way down a flight of stairs and, after a short walking about, I discovered the mess where lunch was being served and joined the lineup. Inside, I discovered a small, narrow room, wide enough to hold a table and benches for the stewards and seamen, lit by a single porthole.

I met up with Bill, and we exchanged comments on our morning activities. We were joined by two other cabin stewards, Bob Ferguson and Sandy Bryce.

As I entered the mess, I looked around and noted several ship-like features: the table was anchored to the deck to avoid movement in rolling seas; the benches alongside were moveable; along the edge of the dining table was a wooden ledge, that would prevent plates, cups, and condiments from sliding off during rough seas; and the menu listing two selections, plus a beverage and dessert, was written on a chalkboard. In short, the mess and furniture were utilitarian, easy to keep clean, and suitable for seas of any nature.

There was one sitting for lunch, where we had an opportunity to share our stories and observations. On this occasion, all of us cabin boys sat as a group, exchanging information and becoming better acquainted. While I felt that it would take me a long time to get to know everyone, it was sure to be an interesting voyage.

As we finished our lunch, the chief steward approached and instructed us to bring our cleaning and waxing equipment to the dining salon.

The dining salon was located on the forward area of the Promenade Deck. This large, bright room at the bow of the ship had panorama windows stretching from starboard to port. Judging from its appointments, it was intended for the captain, officers, the medical team, and invited dignitaries.

Before we could wash and wax the linoleum floor, we had to move the tables and chairs into one section of the room. Several seamen assisted us in this job. After one section was dry, we moved the furniture there and set to cleaning the remaining dirty area. It was a time-consuming task that had to be completed in time for preparations of the evening meal.

The chief steward kept a close eye on us, instructing us as to how we must do the cleaning and waxing, issuing a constant stream of observations as to spots we'd missed. We quickly took our cue from the seamen who ignored the chief's directions and continued regardless.

In the end, the job was deemed a success. At least, the chief did not point out any slips of the mops. We had been under the gun, so to speak, but the back and forth comments and bantering among us made the job easier. It was clear that, as a group, we were developing an element of camaraderie.

We then were instructed to wash and wax four passenger cabins and both companionways on the Promenade Deck, the latter three times. The chief steward informed us that the Promenade Deck was reserved exclusively for the passengers. The logic of this statement escaped me, but I took my cue from the seamen who had worked with us in the salon and paid scant heed to this message.

Once again, we bent to our tasks and soon discovered that the companionways were in need of a thorough cleaning. However, we could only do one companionway at a time and the third coat of wax took much longer to dry than the first two. Oh, well, I thought, it would take a lot of elbow grease to remove the wax the next time this job was done.

In the end, everything was shipshape—all spiffed up and ready for the arrival of the passengers.

It was late in the day and our work was finished when the chief steward approached us. "Go and get your bags and follow me," he ordered. We gathered up our few belongings and followed the chief steward downstairs to the lower decks. It seemed as though any hope of being assigned the posh digs shown upon arrival were being dashed. We followed him down yet another set of stairs to the depths of the ship and the Main Deck, where the air was quite warm and hummed with constant noise. We were definitely either close to, or below the waterline.

"This is your cabin," the chief said, pointing to a door. Inside, we stared at a cramped space with four bunk beds and lit by a single light dangling from the ceiling. With that, the chief left us.

We tossed our bags into a corner and sat on the lower bunks. For a few moments, we sat in silence as we took in our new home. It was obvious this cabin had been used for storage. It had not seen a mop or broom for a long time, if ever. The only source of fresh air came from a small vent over the cabin door. Almost in unison, we expressed our displeasure. It didn't help, either, knowing that the French-speaking cabin boys were nicely tucked into posh living quarters two decks above us on the Promenade Deck. Talk about steerage. We were right next to the engine room.

I chose an upper bunk, with its head close to the air vent. This way, I would get the fresh air first, I thought.

Next, we decided to utilize our new-found cleaning talents. We removed the junk that had been stored there, then with mops, brooms, and other cleaning materials got to work. Soon, the stale odour that had filled our nostrils upon arrival was replaced with fresh scents of soap and water. We were pleased with its spic-and-span transformation. It was almost livable. "We were well trained by our mothers," Bob Ferguson joked.

"Speak for yourself, I'm still in training!" exclaimed Sandy Bryce.

As we sat around on our beds, the laughter and banter continued as we talked over the day's events. We decided to name our cabin "The Black Hole of Calcutta," in reference to the small dungeon at Old Fort William in Calcutta, India, where, in 1756, more than a hundred British prisoners of war died in the space of a single night. Even though we had done an expert job at cleaning, there was nothing we could do to change its overall state, hence the name. However, we all felt better after we had finished cleaning and proceeded to square away our personal belongings. Adding personal touches helped to lessen the meanness of our living quarters.

After our evening meal, we went up to the Promenade Deck and took in the sights and sounds of busy Montreal Harbour. The Royal Yacht *Britannia* was tethered to a quay not far from the *Howe*. Nearby, there were naval destroyers from the United States and Canada. The Queen and Prince Philip had arrived in Canada to participate in the Opening Ceremonies of the St. Lawrence Seaway, along with other dignitaries, including the President of the United States, Dwight D. Eisenhower, and Prime Minister John G. Diefenbaker.

This was my first visit to Montreal. I had heard rumours of the type of nightlife one might experience in this large cosmopolitan city, and we were curious to see for ourselves if the city lived up to its reputation. As the weather was warm, we dressed in light summer clothes and casually set out from the ship seeking adventure. We toured the port area, but it was too early to witness anything "notorious." So much for wicked activity. After a few hours of walking and taking in the sights, we returned to the ship.

"I'm too pooped to pop!" I exclaimed as we entered our cabin. The others agreed with me. We soon tucked ourselves into bed and turned out the light.

Although I was very tired, a myriad thoughts raced through my head, including my cabin mates—Bill Kendall, with whom I'd driven from Ottawa, Sandy Bryce, and Bob Ferguson.

Sandy Bryce, also from Ottawa, was about six feet tall, slim, with dark brown hair. He had a pleasant face that matched his demeanour. He enjoyed discussions and was quick to share a joke. He was a friendly, likeable chap who expressed his feelings, and I thought we would get along just fine.

Bob Ferguson was from southwestern Ontario. He was about five-feet-eight with brown hair and a ready smile. However, behind that smile, there was sure to be some skulduggery in the planning stages. He liked to party, yet had a serious side to him as well. The eldest of us four, he could be counted on for good counsel.

Before long, my mind shut down and the shades of sleep drifted over me. My last conscious thought was of waking up to face another very busy day on the morrow.

After breakfast the next day, we were assigned to clean two communal latrines, located mid-point on the Promenade Deck. I noted how convenient they were from both the port and starboard sides of the deck. I considered this an important piece of information should the ship encounter heavy seas.

In the meantime, it was evident on first glance that the latrines were in dire need of heavy duty cleaning. The true communal nature of the latrines made itself known to one's olfactory senses. It took a lot of time and elbow grease to return these facilities to a state of freshness and cleanliness.

Suddenly, the klaxons blared throughout the ship. We had no idea what this alarm meant, but its loudness and persistence indicated possible danger. The seamen rushing past us said that it was a signal for all crew, including cabin boys, to go immediately to the ship's lifeboat stations.

When we arrived at our assigned station on the aft section of the Boat Deck, we donned our life jackets. Although fat and uncomfortable to the point that they limited mobility, we knew how important they would be if we were ever in a serious situation at sea. I recalled reading a novel about sailors whose ship had been torpedoed in the North Atlantic during the Second World War, prompting sailors to jump into the freezing cold waters where survival time was short. This was a sobering thought as we went through what would be the first of several lifeboat drills.

The lifeboat was well secured to davits with lines and pulleys for lowering the boat into the water. It appeared as though the operation of this equipment was beyond the skills of rookie cabin boys. Fortunately, the seamen at the station explained the mechanics involved in preparing the lifeboat for launching. When the locking devices were released, the lifeboat could slide down the davit rail to the edge of the deck. Then the canvas cover was removed from the boat, meaning the boat was in a position to be loaded with passengers. We were then instructed on how to secure the lifeboat to the ship. By the end of the drill, I questioned my ability to step into the breech should there be a real emergency instead of a drill.

Next came the fire drill. Our station was No. 14 on the aft portion of the Promenade Deck, just below the Boat Deck. Our instructions for assisting the crew stationed here proved a sobering experience. Although I paid special attention to all the intricacies of this exercise, I feared that I would not remember all the details. Fortunately, the seamen were experienced and demonstrated that they had the necessary skills.

I couldn't help but think of that fateful first and last voyage of the RMS *Titanic*. It had only been a few months since I had studied E.J. Pratt's epic poem *The Titanic* in English class, a chilling tale. It was a given we would encounter icebergs on our voyage.

The last job of this busy day was to clean the Eskimo Quarters. We were sent to a hold in the bow of the ship, access to which was through a hooded doorway and passageway of stairs down to a lower deck. The stairway, although short, was dark. I felt like

I was descending into the ship's brig. The quarters comprised a room of steel walls, ceiling, and floor, all painted a dull grey and equipped with bunk beds and latrines. It was smaller than what I had imagined a hold to be. We later discovered that our Eskimo passengers had the initiative to enjoy each others' company regardless of their surroundings.

Of course it was dirty, having been unoccupied since the previous summer's voyage, and our task was to make it clean. The Eskimos were returning home after being treated for tuberculosis at sanitariums in Montreal and Hamilton. We gave the hold a thorough cleaning and were pleased with the results of our labour. We hoped it would pass inspection by the chief steward.

"You fellows have certainly done a good job here," Chief Steward Moreau commented. "I am sure our guests will be happy. The clean surroundings will make their trip home more enjoyable."

We had again struck a favourable chord with our boss. I hoped the message that we gave our all to assigned tasks got around the ship.

There was a hum aboard the ship. Something momentous was happening. Several crew members hurried about completing last-minute tasks. Breakfast was eaten quickly. We were facing another busy day, as the ship was preparing to sail.

Orders from the bridge directed seamen as the ship's barges were hoisted aboard and secured to the decks. Below decks, the engines emitted loud rumbling sounds that vibrated throughout the ship, and the lines securing the ship were cast off. It was mid-morning on Saturday, June 27, 1959, as the *Howe* slowly slipped away from the quay and turned towards the open waters of the St. Lawrence River. Destination: Quebec City.

Shortly after leaving the mooring, we heard the "wop-wop" sound of a helicopter. It hovered over the stern of the ship and gently landed under many watchful eyes. The seamen secured the helicopter to the deck as the blades slowed to a stop. The pilot and engineer made a point of greeting all who watched. For me, this was very special. I had never been this close to a helicopter before. Another new experience.

Daily general duties for the cabin boys included making up the passenger cabins, which were used by the medical staff. Each cabin contained two bunks with curtains and a small washroom with sink and toilet. The beds were anchored to the ship's bulkheads, making it awkward to make the bed, particularly when the linen had to be changed. The floors of each cabin were swept daily, and washed and waxed weekly. Each cabin boy was responsible for a number of cabins. Occasionally, due to their irregular hours, a member of the medical staff would still be in bed when we were on our rounds, meaning that the making up of these cabins would have to be delayed.

We also had duty in the pantry, which was located off the dining lounge. It was not a large area, making it a bit of a squeeze to move around. Access to the pantry was through a swinging door to the dining salon and another door leading to the passageway on the starboard side. It had a large sink for washing dishes and a countertop for drying them. There was also counter space for small electrical appliances, as well as a large coffee urn. Above the counters hung several cupboards for storage. The stewards could prepare light meals or snacks here, as well as coffee and tea. Overnight, the night waiter was stationed here to prepare light meals and beverages for those on shift.

One deck below the pantry/salon was the galley, where the main meals were prepared. Meal orders were given to the stewards who sent them to the galley below. Food was delivered to the pantry via a dumbwaiter, where the stewards plated the food before serving it to the diners.

During my first shift in the pantry, my orders were to wash and dry by hand the dishes, cutlery, and utensils throughout the meal. As soon as I had washed, dried, and stored a number of these items, the stewards would collect them and serve newly seated passengers and officers. After two-and-a-half hours of dishwasher duty, I had cleaned, dried, and stored the last plate and utensil, ready for the next meal.

There were also two stewards in the pantry, Louis and Armand, who were responsible for waiting on the tables in the salon.

"You will be working with these men," the chief advised me. "They have been on this trip before, so they are familiar with the accepted manner of doing the job." With that said, the chief left and Steward Louis took over. He carefully explained his job expectations. What could be simpler?

"You have to wash the dishes, dry the dishes, and put them away. But, remember: you must always have clean dishes and cutlery ready for use up until the last guest leaves the salon." Steward Armand looked on, nodding his head in agreement and carefully watching for my reaction.

Very quickly, Steward Louis made clear that he was a stickler for orderliness and cleanliness, traits well suited for the job. As I stood there listening as he pointed out the locations for storing dishes, glasses, and cutlery, as well as the pots and pans, I observed that he was a thin man, who stood about six feet, with dark hair and a thin face that showed little emotion. While he was all business on this occasion, I soon learned that he could be obsequious—a "yes man"—somewhat like Uriah Heep in Charles Dickens' *David Copperfield*.

In the pantry, Steward Louis scurried about like the White Rabbit in *Alice in Wonderland*. While I don't recall him ever looking at a pocket watch and saying, "I'm late, I'm late, for a very important date!" he never stopped. Was it any wonder we cabin boys nicknamed him "Leaping Louis," or later, the Leaper!

Steward Armand, on the other hand, was a man of few words, and those mostly in French. However, he carried out his duties quietly and efficiently. During our first meeting, I perceived that he was pleased to meet me, but behind those eyes, I saw a bit of mystery, which piqued my curiosity. We nicknamed Steward Armand, "The Bass," as his lower jaw, when viewed in profile, appeared to extend beyond his upper jaw, similar to the fish of the same name.

By 8 p.m., the tasks in the pantry had been completed, so I went out on deck. The fresh breeze was a relief after the stale air of the cramped pantry. We were approaching Quebec City, and I could see the Quebec Bridge and Wolfe's Cove. I was fascinated and tried to imagine the difficulties that had faced General Wolfe as he and his troops stormed the cliffs to capture the Quebec fortress 200 years before. The lush shoreline of early summer turned my thoughts to my family who were spending the holiday weekend at the lake. A wave of homesickness came over me as I thought of them in familiar surroundings, enjoying swimming, boating, and other water activities. I had only been on the ship a few days, but it seemed as though an age had passed since I had left home. However, my thoughts quickly returned to the present at the prospect of going ashore to tour the city.

The main feature of interest was La Terrasse, a long, wide boardwalk adjacent to the renowned Château Frontenac. From this vantage, one could look down on the Old City. It was a well-known rendezvous for sailors (including those from U.S. Navy ships also in port) who sought the company of *les jeunes filles*. And sure enough, there were many young ladies, dressed in their summer finery, out strolling along the boardwalk. Laughing and chatting in French amongst themselves, it appeared as though they were sharing unflattering comments on the choice of men available. The pointing of fingers at selected men accompanied by laughter was perhaps a means of luring some to venture into a conversation, or *je ne sais quoi*.

We sat down on one of the many park benches placed at intervals along the boardwalk and observed with interest the variety of activities going on about us. The girls, the buildings, the panoramic view—it was all captivating.

On Sunday, June 28, the ship departed Quebec City. The day dawned cool, rainy, and foggy. We cabin boys set to finish cleaning all the cabins in preparation for the last remaining passengers to board, the medical staff.

After our midday meal, I joined my cabin mates washing the walls of the Second (upper) Deck and the Main (lowest) Deck. The Second Deck was not too difficult to clean; however, the Main Deck, which included the engineers' section, was very dirty, requiring much elbow grease, soap, and hot water.

Our next destination was a slow down rather than a scheduled stop, at Father Point (*Pointe-au-Père*), Rimouski. Since Montreal, the *Howe* had been under the command of a pilot, as per shipping regulations for all vessels sailing on inland waters. His services were no longer required and he was about to disembark. The small motorized craft that was approaching would take him back to shore. In addition to dropping the pilot, this was the last opportunity for mail to go out. This was a wake-up call for me. The last mail! I hurried to get another letter written to go ashore.

The *Howe* set course down the St. Lawrence River and into the Gulf of St. Lawrence. I observed that there was a notable increase in the size of the waves and force of the wind. The ship took on a distinct rock-and-roll motion, which made me dizzy. Down below in our cabin, I put my hand on the side of the ship, and I could feel the sea water splashing against the hull. Freshly laundered clothing, hanging from the cabin ceiling, swayed back and forth. The weather had changed, and I wondered how the ship would ride in heavy seas. I also wondered if I would be seasick.

I had made friends with the quartermaster, a liaison to happenings on the Bridge. I found him a reliable source of information. My head was filled with many questions as to the operation of the ship. I enjoyed chatting with him as he answered many questions. According to him, rough weather was predicted by late evening and into the next day.

He asked if I had my "sea legs," yet. I would find out very soon.

# Chapter Three

# Northward Bound

We seldom saw the night waiter, Jacques Joli-Coeur, as his shift ended at 6:30 a.m., but we certainly were aware of his existence. His last duty was to awaken us with a loud knock on our cabin door and the words, "Time to rise and shine boys," or "Up an' at 'em!" There were many times we did not appreciate this service, but we could not roll over and ignore it.

Our daily routines were quickly established. Cabins had to be made up and duties attended to in the pantry. Additional duties were assigned by Chief Steward Moreau, either by standard operating procedures or by necessity. Although I had not formally toured the ship since joining almost a week before, I had become familiar with many areas through work or a little snooping after hours. By now I was able to locate the necessities to complete the cabin tasks, the special polishing items to clean the brass and portholes, and the pails, wax, and mops required to keep the floors and walls in tip-top shape.

Those areas off my beaten track included the seamen's cabins, the galleys, and numerous mysterious nooks and crannies. Once while off duty, I made a special tour, stopping by the open door of a seaman's cabin. Upon peaking in, I discovered six or seven men squeezed together playing cards. They asked me if I wanted to join in, but I politely refused on the grounds that I did not know the game they were playing. I stayed to watch, and during a break in the play, they asked me many questions as to my background. They noted that my last name, "Ault," was usually a suffix for francophone names. I explained the historical background of my name (from the Anglo-Saxon for "old") and linked the history behind the name to the opening of the new Seaway (Ault Island

and Aultsville were both submerged during the recent flooding). This prompted more questions and lengthy answers. Too soon I had to take my leave, along with some new friendships.

I quickly discovered the tuck shop and the postmaster's office, both important as a visit to them meant a chance to chat and learn more about what made the ship tick.

I also considered the postmaster an important person to know, as I viewed postal communications as critical. To pass the time off duty, I would write to my parents, whom I knew would share my letters with my siblings, my grandmother, and several aunts, uncles, and cousins. I also wrote many letters to my girlfriend. I did not think I was homesick, but I wanted to maintain my connection with home and there were times of quiet contemplation during which I felt very much alone.

The postmaster would let me know when the mail could leave the ship, occasions that were few and far between. His friendly demeanour made it easier to accept the fact that my letters would sit in his office as part of a growing pile for possibly weeks on end, before actually winging their way to designated recipients.

He was a tall man with bushy dark hair and wrinkles, who commanded a wealth of knowledge combined with experience. His round, ruddy face seemed always to be lit with a smile. He made me feel comfortable from the start, and always had time to answer my questions. He also allowed me to frank some of my own letters, which was probably quite irregular and against all regulations, but I surmised my honest face convinced him to trust me.

The franking tool was a small, hammer-like implement with an engraved metal head that had a small, wheel-like item for changing the date. I did not hesitate to accept when he first offered me the opportunity to frank a letter, but I did not want to make a mistake with Her Majesty's Mail and get in trouble with the Queen.

"Just take the hammer," he explained, "hit the ink pad, then hit the envelope. Be sure to frank the postage stamp so that it cannot be reused." It took skill to make sure the post mark was clearly visible, but I am sure that Postie could do this without giving it a second thought.

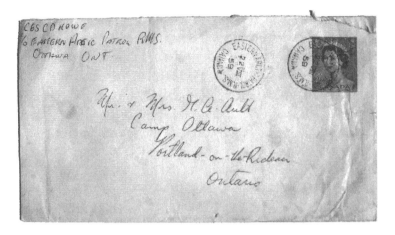

*An envelope I franked in the postmaster's office. Author's collection.*

The tuck shop was operated by Chief Steward Moreau and was open in the early evening, just after dinner on Mondays, Wednesdays, and Saturdays. Like a kid in a candy shop, I would gaze at the variety of candies, gum, and other tasty delights available for purchase. The tuck shop had a wide assortment of personal care items for sale as well. Sometimes we would go to the tuck shop to purchase popcorn just before going to see the featured movie. This was the chief steward's special project, and I speculated that, by the end of the voyage, he would have made a tidy profit.

The tuck shop gave me opportunity to chat with the chief in a relaxed atmosphere, and it was during these visits I discovered another side of my boss. He was concerned that the cabin stewards treated all the passengers well. Not only did our good work make him shine in the eyes of the passengers, but also the other officers. I was certain the members of the medical team expressed their praises, and I felt better after having these chats.

During breakfast in the mess one day, the chatter around the table focused on our progress northward as well as our tasks for the day. The chief steward had outlined our work schedule a few days before, which was based on an eight-hour day. Any additional work could be assigned with the incentive of possible overtime pay. That day, I was assigned to duties in the pantry, which, in my eyes, was more of a scullery—a room in which dishwashing and other kitchen chores were done.

There seemed to be an endless stream of people strolling in for breakfast, including senior officers, followed shortly thereafter by medical staff. I was kept busy washing and drying dishes, as even more crew and passengers arrived in the dining salon for their morning meal. The pile of dirty dishes grew higher, no matter how hard I tried to keep up.

Afterwards, we set to cleaning the cabins, which extended into the afternoon. On this day, we were assigned to clean the Eskimo quarters.

The Eskimo quarters were located in the forward section of the ship, which was prone to extreme movement during storms. The ship was sailing into stronger winds and higher seas, causing the Eskimos to be seasick from the ship's irregular movements. Their constant groans and frequent trips to the latrines (not everyone made it in time) proved beyond doubt they were in extreme discomfort. Their possessions, although meagre, had become dislodged and were tossed haphazardly about their living quarters. In short, the place was a mess, and our job was to thoroughly clean it. The Eskimos had smiles and lots of "EEEs" all around as they expressed their joy and thanks for the sparkling clean living quarters.

We passed Seven Islands[1] about noon, with Anticosti Island slipping by our starboard after nine that evening. We were now in the Gulf of St. Lawrence. The weather was cool and windy with gusts of wind around twenty to thirty knots. The waves continued to increase in size, and storm warnings were issued for the area. It promised to bring a great deal of discomfort to those of us who had not yet acquired the coveted sea legs. The *Howe* was a small ship: 295 feet in length and 50 feet in breadth with a shallow draft. It was likened to a wood chip on a very large body of turbulent water. The bow and stern would bob up and down, followed by the sideways rolling from port to starboard, then back again.

I welcomed the opportunity to go to bed early. Once lying down, the nausea seemed to lessen. I had not experienced any

---

1  Sept-Îles, Quebec.

vomiting, but there had been some tense moments. I managed to get a good night's sleep.

Upon waking the next morning, I lay in bed and planned my tasks for the day. It was necessary to continue with the assigned tasks, yet be prepared to rush to the head and not create more mess to clean up.

Why eat? I knew full well I would lose everything in short order. Seasickness is no fun. It weakens you. Your only desire is to go to bed and sleep. In a prone position, the nausea eases.

I decided to go out on the Promenade Deck and hopefully get some fresh air. The sky was overcast and dense fog surrounded us, making it difficult to determine where the grey sea ended and the grey sky began. Closer to the ship, I was amazed by the sight of large waves, capped with fierce, white spumes. I looked up at the mast above the Bridge. The ship was rolling through many degrees off-centre, and I questioned how close the cross-spar could get to the water before disaster struck. I hung firmly onto the rails, wondering as to whether the ship would recover, or just keep on rolling. As oncoming waves crashed over the bow, pouring large quantities of water onto the forward deck and down amidships into the scuppers, I feared the ship would be swamped.

Back and forth, and up and down, followed by more trips to the head. There was nothing else to do but to ride out the storm.

We also had assigned tasks to complete. The cabins were attended to and put in shape, albeit in a hasty fashion. On pantry duty, I had to be relieved to visit the head, although by now I had nothing left to bring up—just dry heaves. While on deck I could obtain some relief, down in the cramped, stuffy, and windowless pantry, the nausea intensified. Fortunately, one of the members of the medical staff, on hearing of my plight, gave me a "grab all" (Gravol). I went to my cabin for some rest and let the pill do its work. Later, I arose feeling a little better and had a light lunch of dry bread, baked veal, potatoes, and turnip without any butter or gravy. I was indebted to the seasoned sailor who suggested the menu. I ate at the captain's table. Although he had long ago eaten his meal, a feeling of superiority crept over me as I enjoyed my cure for seasickness at his table.

Shortly thereafter, we were assigned further duties of "passing the mop" over the walls and floors of the passageways.

(The term "passing the mop" was used by the chief steward; it was a rough translation from the French into English. In no time, the other two stewards picked up the phrase with a mischievous twinkle in their eyes, and it became a colloquialism among us. For instance, we would quote Steward Leaping Louis when out of earshot with, "We make the overtime and pass the mop!" followed by gales of laughter.)

Suddenly, there was a deep blast from a horn, followed by several more, which echoed throughout the ship. I'd never heard it before, but I soon learned it was the foghorn, sounded as a warning to other ships possibly sailing nearby. The *Howe* had passed another ship in the Strait of Belle Isle, but the weather was worsening, with visibility reduced to zero and reports of ice spotted on radar, all of which gave rise to additional fearful concerns. The foghorn maintained its regular blasts throughout the night and into the next day. The forecast for the next day, July 1, was more of the same. Shipboard life had taken on a new dimension.[2]

More icebergs were sighted in the morning as the ship continued to sail slowly northward. One, I estimated, was about half a mile long and about 1,000–1,500 feet high. It was quite a sight, and I recalled E.J. Pratt's description of icebergs in his epic poem, *The Titanic*. I retrieved my camera from the cabin so as to capture an image of my first iceberg sighting. This one, just off the ship's beam, threatened to do serious, life-threatening damage if we approached any closer. As we sailed by, I was convinced that such an iceberg could easily rip through the steel skin of a ship and send it to a watery grave.

It was overcast and rainy with visibility of about five miles. We were surrounded by ice, either as pack ice or "growlers," which are small chunks of ice. There were thirty-seven icebergs reported in the vicinity of our sailing course.

July 3 dawned warmer and fog lifted by afternoon, as the sun tried to break through the clouds. The winds had decreased and,

2   Looking over my diary, I was hoping I had made some reference to Dominion Day. After all, it was a statutory holiday. However, there was no celebration of Canada's ninety-second birthday, not a hint of the importance of this historic day.

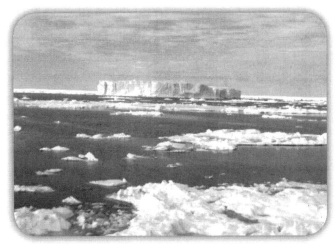

*Iceberg surrounded by growlers. Author's collection.*

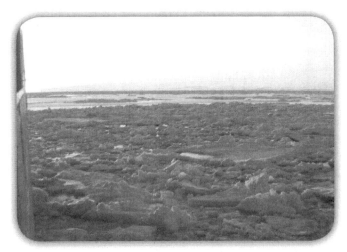

*Photo taken from Starboard Promenade Deck in evening.*
*Author's collection.*

with pack ice around us, the sea was calm. A welcome break from the rough seas earlier in the week. We were making good time travelling about eleven knots per hour.

The quartermaster, Mr. Barbeau, kept us up to date as to the latest news from the Bridge when our paths crossed on deck. We considered this as our own individual pipeline to important and vital information and that our friendship with Barbeau entitled us to this insight into the inner workings of the ship. Little did we realize at that time that the information was recorded as part of the ship's sailing log. At any rate, it was an opportunity to expand friendships and tap into a source of information.

Quartermaster Barbeau was an interesting and friendly person, with a pleasant face and demeanour, which made him very approachable. His smile opened most conversations, and it was soon evident that he had many years of experience at sea travelling in the North. He steered the ship.

As the crew were finishing their supper, the boat drill horns sounded. I had just taken a shower and was in the midst of getting dressed, so was forced to leave for my station wearing only a cotton T-shirt and trousers. Was it ever cold on deck, but it was just a quick drill, I thought, so would soon be able to get back down below.

We scrambled to our assigned stations where we were joined by a few seamen. While shivering uncontrollably, I tried to recall the instructions learned at the last drill, particularly the sequence and required procedures at each step. What if the seamen tested our memory to recall what we had learned previously? My mind was a blank. Much to my relief, the seamen took the lead as they instructed us in additional tasks—the many steps in preparing and lowering the lifeboat. Too much information, however; I did not think I could ever remember the sequence, let alone be responsible for the actual lowering of the boat safely.

The officers timed us as we completed the drill. We must have received a passing grade from the senior officers who inspected us, as we were then sent to our respective fire stations. There was a lot to learn, and procedures were explained in detail. This was a serious drill and everyone paid close attention, but I could hardly wait to return to the cabin. Finally, the drills were over and we were dismissed. I immediately went to our cabin, dressed in warm clothes, and crawled into bed.

I was unable to get to sleep, however, so I put on even more warm clothes and went up to the Promenade Deck. It was late in the evening, but the sun did not set until around 9:45 p.m., so there was still sufficient light to take in the sight of large ice packs and growlers. I had an opportunity to have a chat with Dr. Lane, the ship's radiologist, who was also taking a turn on the deck. Back in my cabin, I reflected on our conversation, where we had shared stories of family and home, and began thinking about my family. We had not been at sea for long, having only recently left Quebec City, but it had been more than two weeks since I said goodbye to my family in Ottawa. I realized I missed them and longed for communication from them.

After our evening meal the next day, no sooner had we settled on our bunks in our cabin to chat about our experiences of the day, there was a knock on the door. Upon opening the door, there stood Quartermaster Barbeau.

"May I come in and join you?" he asked.

We invited Barbeau in and he sat down on one of the lower bunks.

"I guess you are wondering why I came to visit?" Most definitely. Was this a social visit or something else?

Barbeau commented that he wanted to share stories of the North, some amusing, some less so.

We listened intently as Barbeau spun his tales. One involved charts being mixed up, while another featured a long length of chain that had somehow become entangled around a ship's rudder. The solution was to send two seamen into the freezing water to free the chain from the rudder. He explained the dangers these men faced and the consequences to the ship should the attempt to free the rudder fail. Fortunately, the rudder was freed and the men returned safely to the ship.

Now, we were making our own adventures and hopefully we would know how to avoid those situations that may be fraught with trouble. Regardless, he assured us that we would have stories to tell when we returned home.

Barbeau looked around our cabin and noticed a photograph of my girlfriend, Liz. This treasured memento was taped to the bulkhead over my bunk. As I lay in bed, I could look up and be reminded of my gal back home. Liz was wearing a pretty floral dress that she had worn on one of our special dates. Her warm smile was a delight.

"Who is that very pretty girl?" he asked.

"That is my girlfriend." I hoped that a curt answer would prevent further comments.

"*C'est si bon!*" exclaimed Barbeau. "She is very beautiful!"

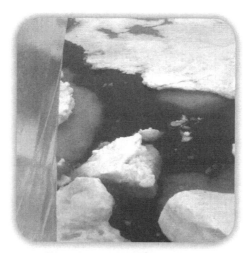

*Photo taken while leaning over the bow starboard rail. The ship was completely surrounded by ice. Author's collection.*

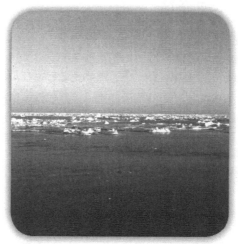

*Photo taken before sunset of the ice surrounding Acadia Cove near Resolution Island. Author's collection.*

He continued with his praises of how lovely she looked, followed by more statements of adoration. Did he have a crush on her? He threatened to have me dropped off at Grise Fiord. Was he serious?

Later that evening, a large ice pack was sighted off the port bow, as well as growlers and three icebergs. The speed of the ship was reduced, to the point where we were just puttering along, slowly and cautiously, through the huge ice floes.

These floes were considered a potential danger to the ship.

While we had to negotiate the floes with care, it was still quite a sight. The ship was completely surrounded by ice. Looking out from the deck over the wide expanse of the ice pack, I could not see any open water. There must have been a lot of activity on the Bridge under these conditions. The Arctic forgave no mistakes.

At noon the next day, our position was about twenty miles from Resolution Island. The temperature remained cold, and it was foggy with limited visibility. The ship was unable to get any closer to the island, and thus we circled, waiting for the ice and fog conditions to improve.

We arrived in Acadia Cove at Resolution Island at 6 p.m. on July 4. The ship had had to crash through floes from three miles offshore, in order to create a safe passage. The noise emitted during this exercise was like something I had never heard before, as if something was being destroyed. Impact with one very large floe caused the entire ship to shudder from bow to stern. In our cabin located deep in the belly of the ship, the rocking of the ship caused the upper bunks to sway back and forth. I was up in the bow to watch the ship crash through the ice floes, when the ship came to a dead stop. Were we in for it now? Was this one of those misadventures, such as Barbeau had told us? Were we stuck solid in the ice?

"Reverse engines!" the Bridge ordered.

There was a loud and unfamiliar cranking sound as the engines were put into reverse, causing the entire ship to shudder. I feared another thrust forward to break the ice would rock the entire ship and flip me over the side into the icy sea.

I left my observation perch in the bow of the ship and took up a safer post, mid-ship on the Promenade Deck. As I looked over the side railing, sure enough, I saw eddies of sea water and bubbling white froth from under the ship, proof that we were going backward. Ice chunks squirted out from under the forward portion of the ship.

All was suddenly quiet.

Then the engines, deep inside the ship, rumbled loudly as full power was delivered to the ship's propellers, pushing the ship forward. The ship crashed into the ice once again, riding up on the big, thick floes. The weight of the ship cracked the floes, which I could see sliding out from under the bow. Back and forth the *Howe* continued in such a manner, gradually making headway through the ice. I hung on to the ship's railing to steady myself. I learned later that the ship was designed to ride up on the ice thus allowing the weight of the ship to break apart the floes, which, as it was early in the season, were thick. Regardless, it was a slow process so as to avoid damaging the ship's steel plates. Back in my cabin, I put my hand on the bulkhead where I could feel the vibrations from the ice floes as they scraped alongside the hull.

Now, THAT was an experience.

From the deck, I could see nothing but ice surrounding the ship. An eerie thought crept into my mind: "Lost in Ice." I knew we were not too far from shore, but the coast was difficult to see. When the fog finally lifted, however, I was presented with quite a sight. This was my first glimpse of northern terrain. Nothing but rocks, hills, snow-filled valleys, and sparse vegetation. I wondered how the Eskimos could survive in this seemingly barren land.

Under normal circumstances, the crew would launch a lighter (motorized barge) to ferry the Eskimos from shore to the ship for their medicals. These were not normal circumstances. Visibility was restricted by fog, and the ice conditions prevented the ship getting close enough to the coast so as to locate a suitable beachhead for landing the barges. As it was not possible to launch the lighters, the helicopter was used to transport the Eskimos, as well as the Department of Transport personnel, from shore. I marvelled at the pilot's skill to take off from and land on the moving ship, as well as fly safely under the poor weather conditions.

Tasks completed, we moved on to our next destination. All reports indicated continued cold temperatures, overcast skies, and ice for the foreseeable future. It appeared as though the ship would have to continue breaking through ice floes.

We were truly in the Arctic now

# Chapter Four

# In the Straits, Part I: Hudson Strait

The next scheduled settlement on the itinerary was Port Burwell, a small community on Killiniq Island, the northeastern tip of land between Ungava Bay and the North Atlantic Ocean. However, steaming across the mouth of the Hudson Strait, the *Howe*'s progress continued to be hampered by heavy pack ice. As it was impossible to sail close to shore, the medical survey and unloading of cargo were delayed.

Our next destination was Wakeham Bay,[3] about halfway up Hudson Strait, but again, the *Howe*'s progress was hampered by pack ice and persistent fog. Sailing at a slow speed, the ship changed course regularly in an attempt to follow the best openings. Waiting for the weather and ice conditions to improve was time consuming, and there was only so much time to complete the patrol's mission.

Shortly after finishing our breakfast, the chief steward approached us. "The medical staff worked through the night. I have been asked by the officer-in-charge to allow them some personal time. Therefore, you will commence your regular duties after the noonday meal."

"Aye, sir," we replied. This was a welcome opportunity to write letters and otherwise relax. We had been at sea for about a week, with all of the accompanying adjustments to new routines, new surroundings, and new faces. This break from the daily routine would give me time to mull over the events that had occurred

---

3 Kangiqsujuaq, Quebec.

since we sailed from Montreal and share thoughts and concerns with my cabin mates.

After lunch, I returned to my regular duties in the pantry. Several of the medical staff were in the salon, dawdling over their lunch, still groggy from lack of sleep, as well as a few guests finishing their coffee. I was anxious to finish my stint in the pantry, when the chief steward approached me.

"You are 'on watch' this afternoon," he said.

"What do you mean, 'on watch'? What are the duties?" While I was familiar with this term as it applied to duty watches on deck, I did not understand how it applied to pantry duty.

"You must sweep the salon floor, serve tea or coffee and snacks to the ship's officers and passengers, and set the tables for dinner," explained the chief steward abruptly, before he left the pantry.

While I was taken aback with this new duty, I immediately began sweeping the floor. I wanted to get this chore completed before the mid-afternoon break. While I had certainly noticed waiters when dining out in restaurants in Ottawa, I realized I really did not know proper wait staff procedures. Could I perform in the polite and efficient manner the position required?

I soon got the drift of what was expected of me. Passengers who appeared in the salon for their afternoon break kindly directed me as to what they wanted. I took their favourable comments as a sign that I was performing in an acceptable manner and began to relax. Then the captain entered the salon. After he had taken his seat, I approached him and requested his order.

"*Une tasse de café, noir, s'il vous plait. Et frais et chaud.*"

"*Mais oui, tout de suite,*" I replied. Surprised at my quick response—in French—I was glad to have the opportunity to use my limited language skills. I had studied French for many years, but I was still relieved that he had only requested a cup of coffee.

But was it both hot and fresh? Was there plenty in the urn? I dreaded the thought of having to brew another. I did not know how much water and coffee were needed. Fortunately, I was able to prepare the captain's order without any problem and returned to the salon. My hand trembled, however, as I served the captain. Did he notice? I did not know until later that you were to serve from the left and take from the right, but there was an air of informality around him, which was fine by me.

"How are you getting along with your duties?" he asked.

"I am learning each day," I replied. "My cabin mates and the chief steward have been helpful. I am fitting into the routine without any problems." The captain nodded his head. I was dismissed.

Perhaps there was a thaw in our relations, I thought as I mulled over our brief exchange. I had been nervous, fearing that I would say the wrong thing and thereby further tarnishing my reputation in his eyes. I assumed there was nothing untoward, and this brief encounter was not of any major consequence. Then again, there still seemed to be an undercurrent of unease left over from our previous meetings. On second thought, I doubted that any ice between the captain and me was melting. However, I would take care to be always on my toes, to ensure that there would be no further incidents to draw his ire.

I arranged the tables and chairs in preparation for the evening meal, then proceeded to set the tables. Table cloths, cutlery, glasses, cups and saucers, salt and pepper, side plates, and napkins—all items were laid with care and attention to detail. It looked similar to my concept of table settings in a restaurant.

I took my evening meal in the mess and chatted about being "on watch," as well as my encounter with the captain, with my

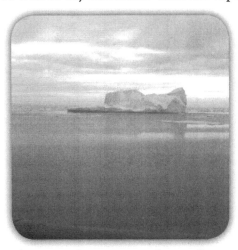

*Iceberg in Hudson Strait. Author's collection.*

fellow cabin mates. The banter around the table put me at ease, and it seemed that it was all smooth sailing ahead. I finished my meal and returned to my duties in the pantry.

Every once in a while, I glanced out the porthole. It was evident the ship was making slow progress, still, and had to buck the pack ice. There were some tense moments as the ship, once again, got stuck in the ice floes. Our noon data, according to the ship's log, placed us at 61° 25′ N Lat. and 67° 07′ W Long.—the middle of Hudson Strait. The sky was overcast, and the ship, with zero visibility, was sailing slowly through the surrounding pack ice at approximately five knots.

As the day advanced, the ice floes cleared, the fog lifted, and visibility improved. Then the sun broke through the clouds and the air suddenly seemed warmer. When we arrived at Wakeham Bay, just east from Cape Hopes Advance, at 9:15 p.m., the sun was still high in the sky.

However, no sooner had the ship dropped anchor when a gale force wind, reaching fifty to seventy miles per hour, swept up and over the ship. Surprised by the sudden change, I went out on deck to watch the effects of the wind. I had never experienced such a force.

The ship's crew had already gone into action. They used extra lines to secure the helicopter to the deck, while the helicopter pilot and engineer secured the blades. Anything not tied down was being whipped off the decks and into the sea. The seamen had to lean into the wind and hang on to whatever was solid to avoid being blown over the side as well. Then, as quickly as the wind had swept up it was gone, leaving a calm behind. Another mystery of the North.

The settlement of Wakeham Bay, while small, was picturesque. Impressive rock formations rose up on either side of the bay, while nestled below were three shacks, two sheds, and five tents. The number of Eskimos in this community was estimated around a hundred, so the medical staff would be busy. Throughout the day and into the evening, seamen ferried Eskimos to and from the ship by barge. The helicopter transported Eskimos, as well. The captain was anxious to complete the survey as quickly as possible in order to make up time lost due to ice conditions. The ship was scheduled to sail in the morning for Sugluk.[4]

After dinner with pantry duties completed, I went out onto the Promenade Deck for some fresh air and take in the scenery. I met up with Nurse Madeleine Onslow, Dr. Lane (radiologist), Dr. Oschinsky (physical anthropologist), Dave Simpson (hydrographic team), and my cabin mate Bob Ferguson. The conversation was both pleasant and informative, and others soon joined us. This was a happy occasion, a welcome time to socialize. I listened as some individuals offered insights into their personal lives. I knew Dave Simpson from our shared involvement in sports in Ottawa, but the others were relatively new acquaintances. While I felt honoured to be included, I held back at bit, not wanting to come across as outspoken. I felt it was better to be seen and not heard.

The discussion became more serious when the issue of ship morale came up.

"There are some negative aspects regarding the manner in which the captain has shown his bias for a specific language group," observed Dr. Oschinsky. My ears perked up and I started to listen closely. Did this have anything to do with my perceived feelings of frostiness by the captain towards me?

"Some of my colleagues in the medical suite have remarked that they hold the captain in poor regard," commented a nurse. "I have noticed over the past few days, his negative attitude and mannerisms towards us. This has an effect on morale and the cohesiveness of the medical staff." Others from the medical group agreed.

Another nurse spoke up. "There seems to be a noticeable segregation, based on language, during mealtime in the salon. I do not think the captain is aware of this, or at least, he may not see this as a problem. Maybe he will just ignore it?"

Were these seeds of discontent? Too soon the group dispersed.

We were now well into the voyage, and I discovered that I had reached the bottom of my duffel bag: I had run out of clean clothes. This situation had to be remedied. But how? I asked the others how

---

4  Salluit, Quebec.

they washed their clothing. There were no laundry services aboard, at least, not for the crew. While many of the seamen just filled a tub with water and soap and scrubbed vigorously, someone suggested I seek out one seaman in particular, who had fashioned a makeshift washing machine. I sought him out and asked if I could borrow it.

"I use a small garbage pail with a plunger made from a broom handle and a funnel," he explained while instructing me in its use. The funnel had several holes about the size of a penny punched into the flared portion. "It works well. Put warm water into the pail with laundry soap. Make sure the soap is dissolved, then add your clothes. Do not put too many items in the pail at the same time. Then, move the plunger up and down, in an agitator motion. The holes in the funnel make the agitator motion easy. Continue this process until you are satisfied the clothes are clean. Remove the dirty water. Add clean water to rinse the clothes, again using the agitator and the same motion. When you are satisfied, take the clothes out of the water and wring them dry."

I could not wait to use this contraption. I hoped it would work, as I did not want to engage in the labourious task of washing and scrubbing my clothes by hand. I immediately went into the lower galley carrying my clothes, soap, and the newfangled washing machine.

After filling the pail with hot water and detergent, I dumped in my clothes and let them soak for several minutes. Then, I took the plunger and agitated the clothes as instructed. When the water changed from soapy clear to dull grey, I figured my clothes were clean, so I dumped out the dirty water, filled the tub with clean water, then rinsed, again using the agitator. After wringing out the excess water, I hung up my now clean clothes from the ceiling in my cabin to dry. Nothing to it. I was indebted to the seaman who had loaned me his contraption. Worked like a charm.

The next day, Eskimos from the settlement came aboard for their medical checkup. I soon noticed a malodorous odour throughout the ship, which I learned when I ran into an Eskimo boy with Dr. Oschinsky, was a characteristic of the Eskimos. Quite frankly, he stank. However, the three of us had a lively, informative chat with lots of smiles and laughter. The boy had a smattering of English, but there was also an interpreter to assist.

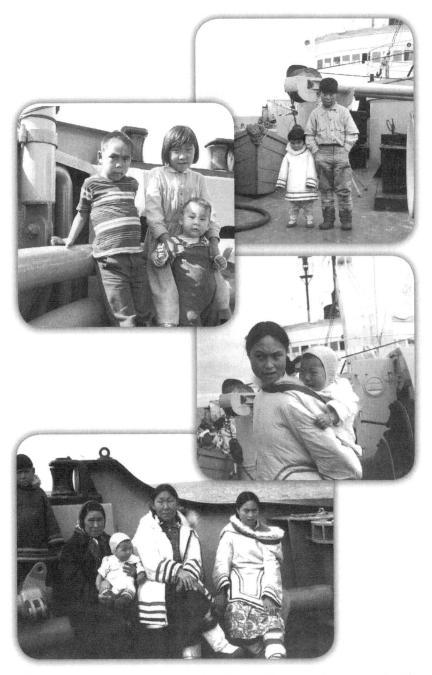

*Photos taken on the bow section of the* Howe. *The young boy pictured with his younger brother may have been the lad I met. Notice their traditional mukluks. Those worn by the boy on the right show evidence that he helps his father. Photos courtesy of Dr. Ruth McLeese.*

The Eskimo were a happy, friendly, independent people, pleased to be aboard the *Howe* during this brief visit. I'm sure they thought we smelled, too.

The Eskimo lifestyle involved hunting and fishing to keep their families fed. The oils from seals, walrus, whales, fish, birds, animals, and other stuff got into their clothes, and therefore was the source of their distinctive odour. Did you think they could take a daily bath? The water temperature only reached a few degrees above freezing during high summer. Perish the thought of washing clothes. They would just freeze when hung out to dry. Hence, their strong odour.

The *Howe* sailed from Wakeham Bay to our next destination, Sugluk. Again, the heavy ice conditions slowed progress, and it was necessary to break a passage with lots of bucking and rocking. I took a break and went out onto the Promenade Deck, where in the distance I could see the dull, grey, rocky coastline interspersed with snow-filled valleys. It all appeared inhospitable, an unwelcome site for those who might want to explore.

After supper, a member of the hydrographic crew approached me on deck.

"I know you are interested in what goes on in our office, in particular, working with hydrographic charts. Would you like to observe the recording of the depths as we approach the anchorage in Sugluk Bay?" he asked.

"Definitely," I responded. "Is there something of special interest?"

"The *Howe* is on course to sail over a shoal," he answered. "We should be nearing this in a few minutes."

I followed the hydrographer below. The Hydrographic Office was about the size of a regular cabin. I had been curious to find out what went on in this busy work station each time I walked past it, and I now could see that it was filled with a variety of electronic equipment, nautical charts, and not to mention desks and chairs.

"Why don't you sit here," he said, pointing to a chair. "You can watch the fathometer as it records the changing depths of water beneath the keel as the ship is sailing."

"Thanks," I responded.

"Nautical charts show that the shoal is thirty feet below the surface of the sea," he informed me. "The *Howe* draws twenty feet."

"Okay," I replied. "That means from the keel to the shoal, there is ten feet of water. Is that not a little close?"

"That's why we are monitoring the ship passing over the shoal. We also record the data to update charts.

"We're confident the ship will clear the shoal, but it will be close," he acknowledged.

Watching the fathometer, I experienced a few tense moments wondering if the information on the charts and the fathometer were accurate. Would the ship sail safely over the shoal? I watched as the recorded depth of the water decreased, and thoughts of imminent disaster raced through my mind. What would happen if the ship ran aground? The ship had been tossed about on the rough seas and punched her way through heavy pack ice. Now this. Moments passed. I held my breath. I heard no sounds of any grinding and crunching. I noticed the fathometer showing the depth of water increasing. As the *Howe* glided over the shoal without scraping bottom or becoming grounded, I breathed a sigh of relief. I was sure the hydrographer beside me did, too.

The *Howe* dropped anchor in the bay opposite the Roman Catholic Mission in Sugluk, a community with ten buildings, two churches, many tents, and a seaplane. It appeared to have a large population. I learned that many Eskimos came for the summer and, undoubtedly, for the *Howe*'s annual visit. A festive-like atmosphere prevailed with our arrival and its promise of needed supplies, building materials, mail, and other special items ordered many months ago.

All signs pointed to a stay that would last for a few days. There was a special breakfast for the medical staff, and from my duty post in the pantry, I predicted that I would be washing dishes late into the morning.

During the day, supplies and cargo were removed from the holds and loaded onto the barges and transported to shore where, with the help of the Eskimos, the cargo was stacked. Some of the cargo would be forwarded to Port Burwell, as ice conditions had prevented the *Howe* from stopping over there. I learned to take opportunities as they arose, an important lesson in the North.

There were barges, the hydrographers' boats, and other landing craft that were launched using the crane on the forward deck. While much of the unloading of supplies proceeded without incident, there were a few tense moments when one of the barges, loaded with barrels of fuel, almost capsized. Also, one seaman was knocked unconscious by a swinging hook. He was taken to the sick bay for medical attention. Just when I thought all was going well, all of a sudden there was an accident. The best advice was to keep your wits about you at all times.

The captain hosted a dinner, the guest list for which included the mission people and representatives of the Department of Transport. This meant there would be more dishes and cutlery to wash and dry. The dinner period would also last longer. Overtime. However, I did not view washing and drying dishes, glasses, and cutlery for several hours a perk. It was seemingly never-ending drudgery.

After dinner, the captain, his guests, senior officers, and medical staff attended impromptu parties throughout the ship.

We heard a first-hand report of one party from Bob Ferguson, who had received an invitation. Lasting by all accounts until the wee hours, it was deemed a success with a good time had by all. Several guests had imbibed copious quantities of alcoholic beverages with the usual outcome. Apparently even the captain was afflicted. This could have explained why he did not show up for breakfast that morning.

Pantry duty required that you stayed on duty until all officers and passengers had finished their meals. As the captain did not show for breakfast during the regular hours of serving, the chief steward made sure I was "on deck" awaiting his arrival. As noon approached, it was time to start prepping for lunch, but still no captain.

"You go and make up your cabins," the chief steward ordered me, "but be sure to return here in time for the regular lunch."

I responded with an, "Aye, aye, sir," and left the pantry to dutifully make up my cabins.

The conversation around our lunch table was interesting.

Bob's retelling and embellishment of the party hijinks of the night before carried the conversation and laughter throughout the meal.

That evening, I, along with my cabin mates, were ordered to go to the Eskimo quarters for cleanup duties. Not a pleasant task. The Eskimos' living habits left much to be desired. It took hard work to clean this area and make it habitable again.

Life in the pantry continued to present a variety of interesting if not amusing vignettes. My shifts there gave me the opportunity to observe standard operating procedures as well as the characteristics of the steward, "Leaping Louis," and his assistant, the waiter Armand we had nicknamed, "The Bass," which provided much fodder for discussion back in our cabin.

The two men often bumped into each other as they attempted to provide timely service to the officers and passengers. As there was little room in the pantry for the three of us to manoeuvre, I did my best to stay well out of their way, all the while trying to keep with the demand for clean dishes and cutlery.

Usually, The Bass referred to me as "my friend," before switching to a rapid *patois*. I was uncertain how to respond. Or, even if I should. Was he really trying to be friends, or was this a sarcastic or derogatory remark aimed at me?

One time, there were practically no clean plates left and Leaping Louis took me to task for my apparent tardiness. Were they blind? I was trying to keep up and was working as quickly as possible.

Later when The Bass called me, "my friend," I ignored him. The atmosphere in the pantry had reached a boiling point. Whose neck was on the block for the next barrage of harsh words? I had my job and I was doing it as best as possible. I knew the two waiters were aware of my mood as they continued chatting with each other.

At one point, The Bass was plating food and dribbled gravy on the edge of the plate. To clean up, he wiped away the offending dribble with his finger and licked it, savouring the tasty juices. In my eyes, this was a disgusting and unsanitary action. Although I found it difficult to tolerate this situation, I refrained from commenting, although I'm sure my displeasure was written all over my face. The Bass got on my nerves, but we had to work together in the close confines of the pantry.

Unbeknownst to Leaping Louis and The Bass, Sandy Bryce and I had studied French language and literature in school. Although our skill in the language was limited, we could understand the gist of their conversations. On several occasions, we heard them talking openly about us in the pantry, and not in a nice way. Their negative comments included character assassination and their perceived notion of what we cabin boys got up to after hours.

I had been outside on deck taking in the sights when I happened to meet up with Kay Denneny and Maddie Onslow, both nurses on the medical team. After a few moments of light conversation, they changed the topic to a more serious note. Armand had recently told them that the chief steward was not pleased with my familiarity with the passengers.

"What?" I exclaimed. "I cannot believe this! Are they spying on me? Are they looking for me to make a misstep?" In all of my personal interactions, both on and off the job, I had considered myself above reproach. I had had no idea that the chief steward thought this way about me, a situation that could result in serious consequences.

Surely he did not believe that my work was below par. Instead, this must be a judgment on how he felt about me personally. Were these and other negative comments falling on the ears of others, besides the nurses? I took this as fair warning, even though in my mind I had not done anything wrong. I and my cabin mates were being watched, and not in a good way.

The ship slipped out of Sugluk just past midnight on a course for Ivujivik.

The settlement's picturesque harbour was inviting with its prominent rocky shoreline. However, no sooner had the *Howe* dropped anchor when the medical survey began and the process of unloading supplies for the community got under way, to be continued throughout the day. The last patient was seen just before the dinner hour.

One event of note was the birth of a child in the early afternoon. Although it was customary for an Eskimo woman to be assisted

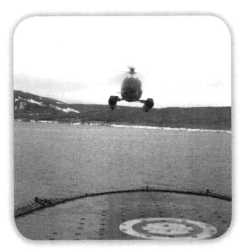

*The Bell helicopter approaching the flight deck. Settlement of Ivujivik in background. Author's collection.*

by other women during birth, the medical officer on board was flown ashore to assist. All went well, and three hours after the delivery, the mother and her child were transported to the ship by helicopter for a checkup, a fortuitous opportunity for them. I was astonished that they were transported to the ship so soon after the birth. I saw this as an example of Eskimos' hardiness.

Every day for the past few weeks, I had been assigned duty in the pantry. I was not complaining, but washing dishes was not my forte. Then, to my surprise, I was informed this was my last day in the pantry and that I had been reassigned to cabin duties.

While I enjoyed swimming and participating in water sports, my hands—in particular my fingers and thumbs—would take on a prune-like appearance from being in the water. If I didn't take care, the skin would open, resulting in wide, open sores. In fact, after weeks of submerging my hands in water, the skin on my fingers and thumbs were scaling away; they were very rough and sore. I had tried wearing rubber gloves, but the condition only worsened. The doctors gave me a special ointment and cotton gloves to ease the pain and relieve the condition, which worked for a while. The cotton gloves also made it difficult to carry out other jobs.

So, my sore hands, plus the tense and uneasy atmosphere in the pantry, made my reassignment a real blessing. I had done my rotation in the pantry, so I foresaw no return to this duty in the future.

We arrived at Cape Dorset about noon on Sunday, July 12. What a beautiful settlement. Pictures do not do it justice. Visible from the ship were many buildings and cabins, and it appeared to be a thriving community. This was confirmed when I discovered Cape Dorset was known as THE centre of Eskimo arts and crafts, many of which have been shipped south over the years for sale to collectors and admirers alike.

Chief Steward Moreau summoned us, the English-speaking cabin boys, to attend an important meeting. He started the meeting by stating there was a serious concern among the senior officers regarding the fraternization between the cabin stewards and the medical personnel. He declared precisely and clearly that, henceforth, we were not allowed to visit the passengers in their cabins. Furthermore, we, the cabin boys, were NOT to invite the passengers to our cabin.

Prior to this edict, we had enjoyed invitations to socialize and visit with members of the medical staff in their cabins. The previous week we had invited Drs. Lane and Oschinsky, as well as the X-ray personnel, Norm Harper and Cort Beckingham, as guests to our cabin. For us, these were special times for relaxation, socialization, and camaraderie.

This pronouncement defined the division between the passengers, who were all anglophones, and the crew, who were all francophones, with the exception of the four English cabin stewards. We saw this as a blatant move to restrict our after-hours activities. The Bridge issued other restrictions, as well: no one was allowed in the Foredeck (bow), or the Poop Deck (stern), and other areas of the ship. They were declared off limits. Finally, the cabin stewards were not allowed to go ashore either by landing barge or helicopter. I did not know of any cabin boy who had gone ashore either by landing barge or helicopter to date. This struck us as an extension of restrictions previously issued to stop any attempt by these persons to go ashore and maybe call Ottawa and place complaints.

Needless to say, we four cabin boys were distressed by these restrictions. In retrospect, they made sense from a safety point of

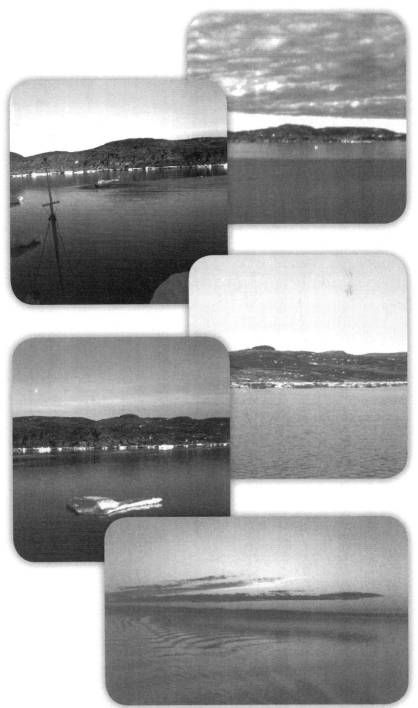

*Cape Dorset at sunset—11 p.m. Author's collection.*

view for the operation, safety, and integrity of the ship. On the other hand, was this a concerted effort to keep the cabin stewards in line?

Word soon got around, resulting in a rising tide of disgruntlement and a lowering of morale. Were the chief steward and Armand the cause? The decision was made to keep our noses to the grindstone, mind our own business, and obey the rules and restrictions. The tension on board, however, could be cut with a knife.

As a group, we expressed our resentment, and after some discussion, we decided to take action. Using the rumour mill, which was obviously very efficient, we would let it be known that we would make phone calls to Ottawa upon arrival at Churchill. Some of us even threatened to leave the ship at Churchill.

In the midst of all this, Ottawa called the ship via the radio phone. The *Howe* was ordered to return to Resolution Island. A mechanic had suffered a heart attack and was in need of emergency medical care.

So much for Plan A.

# Chapter Five

# In the Straits, Part II: Hudson Strait Again

My pictures of Cape Dorset suggest a holiday setting with warm, sun-dappled water and welcoming beaches for sun-seekers. One may easily be carried away with thoughts of those lazy, hazy days of summer so familiar to those of us who live in the south. This illusion is soon shattered, however. This is the North, remember.

I had mixed feelings when I learned that our stay at Cape Dorset was shortened. We would be retracing our steps in order to respond to the medical emergency at Resolution Island, which meant that we might encounter weather and ice conditions similar to those encountered during our initial passage through Hudson Strait. This unplanned trip would also result in time lost for the patrol. The sailing season in the North is short.

It was fortunate, however, that the *Howe* was within short sailing distance of Resolution Island, both in terms of responding to the emergency and hoping to complete the patrol.

As the *Howe* sailed eastward towards Resolution Island, there was a discernible undercurrent of discord, for two reasons: the need to return to Resolution Island, thus foregoing the medical survey at Cape Dorset, and the low morale on board. I and my cabin mates were discouraged by this change in the itinerary.

After lunch, Chief Steward Moreau knocked on our cabin door. This was an unusual occurrence; in fact, it was not in keeping with normal procedures. If he had special tasks for us to perform in the afternoon, he would usually inform us while we were on the job or after the noon meal while we were still in the mess. We assumed the chief had come to our cabin because (a) he wanted to confirm the recent edicts, or (b) because he had important information of specific interest to us. To our astonishment, he outlined a new work schedule. This meant the juggling of cabin assignments and the redistribution of work loads. In addition, Chief Steward Moreau stated that we might be relocated to a cabin on the Promenade Deck. This possibility was hedged in ambiguous terms, leaving us puzzled as to its meaning.

One would think this visit and its accompanying announcements would improve morale below decks. I interpreted it as being akin to rearranging the chairs on the deck of the *Titanic;* an exercise in futility, but interesting just the same. On the other hand, changing cabin assignments opened the door to unsettling the feelings of those passengers who had established favourable working arrangements with their assigned cabin steward, who would by now know their preferences and how to keep their cabin shipshape.

Cabins on the Promenade Deck featured sleeping accommodation for two individuals, an ensuite washroom, a porthole, and interior decoration masking the steel grey walls/bulkheads. We had enjoyed such accommodations for only a few hours when first we boarded, before being assigned to a cabin on the Main Deck two decks below, next to the engine room. The engines operated twenty-four hours a day, emitting a constant thrumming noise. After a few days' residence, we became accustomed to it.

There were four hospital beds with mattresses that carried unsightly evidence of years of use. Two of the beds hung by chains from the ceiling, the two others were firmly secured to the steel floor. The steel walls, ceiling, and floor were painted grey. There was no porthole, and the only fresh air came through an air duct located above the cabin door. The fresh air was a mixed blessing. Yes, it was forced air drawn from outside, but its source was an intake fan located on the top deck behind the ship's funnels. As the engines burned Bunker C fuel oil, the smoke was mixed with particles of soot. In no time, our bedding and clothes were black, so there was some merit to our cabin's original name of the Black Hole of Calcutta. We improvised a filter system for the vent by securing a used nylon stocking, courtesy of the nurses, over the vent opening.

Given time and elbow grease, the cabin eventually took on a somewhat respectable look. While you would not describe it as cozy, even with the addition of some homey touches, it was at least livable and we rechristened it the Executive Suite. A little sarcastic, perhaps, but the name stuck, and was soon referred to as such by others throughout the ship.

The chief steward's announcement that we might be relocated was akin to a declaration of emancipation, a sense of being liberated from the confines of living well below decks. We surmised that our "threat" of the previous day to call headquarters in Ottawa and/or leave the ship at Churchill had found its mark. While it appeared as though there might be some easing up on the new restrictions, we would have to wait and see whether this relocation would, in fact, come into effect.

Forty-eight hours after leaving Cape Dorset, we found ourselves ten miles off Resolution Island. It was shortly after the dinner hour, and the helicopter with a doctor on board left the ship and flew in to the settlement. Visibility had declined, but the pilot was able to locate a safe landing area. The doctor examined the ill mechanic, and then had him loaded onto the helicopter, which then returned to the *Howe*. Once the helicopter was secured to the deck, the captain ordered the quartermaster to adjust the course so as to sail in a westerly direction. Destination: Cape Dorset.

The next day, I went out on deck to catch a glimpse of our surroundings. There was nothing new. The fog had reduced visibility to zero, and the rain fell steadily on the ice surrounding the ship. I looked over the side of the ship, in hopes that I could estimate our speed through this unwelcome mix of poor weather and heavy ice. The faster we went, the larger the bow wave, the greater the splash of water alongside the hull. At least, that was my theory.

Fortunately, by late afternoon, the fog had lifted and the ship was clear of ice. We were back to normal cruising speed.

The next day, as the ship continued on its westerly course, we noticed tension amongst those on board as we made up the cabins. Despite orders, you could not avoid chatting with the passengers while making up their cabins. To exacerbate matters, some fiction had gotten mixed up with the facts, resulting in the only to be expected confusion, upset feelings, and strain.

That evening while below decks in our cabin relaxing after supper, there was a sudden, loud banging on our cabin door. Upon opening, there before me standing in his uniform was First Mate Pelletier. His face was beet red and marked with a scowl that would scare even the staunchest. I did not "know" First Mate Pelletier, as I did not have occasion to talk with him. But I did know that he was determined to get to the bottom of something.

While First Mate Pelletier may have had a jovial side, I never saw it. Unlike other officers, he wore his uniform every day, which he kept spotless. A fastidious man, he had a presence about him, whether he was out and about on deck, or on shore directing the transporting and unloading of cargo. Of average height and build, his mannerisms clearly portrayed him as a man who lived and worked at sea. He was kept busy every day ensuring the Howe was shipshape, and I would oftentimes glimpse him working alongside the seamen.

As the first mate was second only to the captain, or master, I appreciated his no-nonsense approach. He exuded confidence and honesty, and I knew if I approached him with a question about the ship, he would give me a straightforward reply.

But why was he here?

"We have received complaints of a loud, prolonged, boisterous party last evening, which continued into the early morning hours. Do any of you know who was responsible for the disturbance?" Two of our cabin mates had attended a party the previous evening.

"We remained in our cabin, and had no knowledge of this event," said Bill, who had not gone to the party.

There was a moment of silence before the first mate responded. "If there is any other similar occurrence, there will be serious consequences," he threatened as he backed out of the cabin and firmly shut the door.

We knew he was displeased and that he would follow through with "serious consequences." We also knew he knew more than he was letting on.

There was an audible sigh of relief, as we each took a moment to digest what had just happened. At first, nobody dared say anything, then we quietly began discussing all the possible scenarios.

The following day, the medical staff requested that a cabin steward be assigned as an orderly for the ill mechanic, preferably English-speaking. Senior officers selected a francophone, a poor decision in our minds given the level of tension on board and the language spoken by the mechanic. Later, we learned that the nurses agreed with us.

That evening, there was a brawl below decks. Scuttlebutt did not make clear the details, but the dustup followed on the heels of the noisy party of the night before. There may have been some personnel conflicts involving the hydrographers, the ship's crew, and the senior officers. I was unsure of the seriousness of this incident, but it confirmed in my mind that others were also unhappy.

As a consequence, the hydrographers, who had a cabin on the Promenade Deck, were relocated to the Main Deck. In turn, the francophone cabin stewards were moved to the hydrographers' cabin on the Promenade Deck. This turn of events pre-empted the tentative proposal made by Chief Steward Moreau that we might be moved to a cabin on the Promenade Deck. Once again, we were disappointed. We felt we were being treated as second-class citizens.

That evening, the Executive Suite was honoured by a visit from Dr. Oschinsky. He was a jovial man, and we had chatted with him earlier. However, did he know that our cabin was off limits to the passengers? It was doubtful the doctor paid much heed to this rule, as he evidently wanted to discuss the tense situation on board the ship.

Dr. Oschinsky pointed out that the senior officers appeared to be favouring their own—the French-speaking cabin stewards—at our expense. It certainly seemed discriminatory to us. The discussion continued for some time, and each of us had an opportunity to express our own concerns and feelings about the situation.

As we were in the minority, relative to the officers and seamen, the doctor concluded his remarks by stating that we had little choice other than, to quote him, "Eat shit." This situation was character-building, according to the good doctor.

This episode begged the question as to who asked the doctor to chat with us. The passengers relied on the services of the cabin boys. They appreciated the special things done for them. Therefore, to lose the cabin boys at Churchill, not even halfway through the patrol, would raise a red flag in Ottawa, as well as create difficulties in personnel assignments for the remainder of the voyage. Maybe some intervention was required to cool the atmosphere.

We arrived at Cape Dorset around noon the next day. What a great day, with the sun beating down on the calm, blue water. I heard the familiar rattle of the anchor chain as it was lowered and set, so I took a break and went out on the Promenade Deck. Lying off the port beam was a view of this picturesque settlement nestled in a valley of rolling hills. Others had drawn a mental image of the beauty of Cape Dorset before I left Ottawa, and the scene before me lived up to the promise.

Many Eskimos paraded throughout the ship in anticipation of their medical checkup. This must have been a highlight for them, judging by their antics, chatter, and signature, high-pitched "EEEs!" Their infectious laughter cheered our spirits. Who would guess by their clowning and jostling that they were here for a medical.

I was on deck taking in the scenery and watching the activity on board when I saw a young Eskimo boy approach me, carrying a carving and pointing to me. I could see that it was a walrus, lovingly and intricately carved in green soapstone. The boy asked me if I wanted to buy it. There was some negotiation, and we concluded the sale in spite of our language differences. I liked the carving and thought it a good example of the artistic talent at Cape Dorset. However, no sooner had the sale been completed, I was confronted by another Eskimo boy seeking to sell his carving of a seal sitting on a white stone, a replica of an ice floe. The news of a willing buyer must have spread rapidly through the Eskimos on the ship. Again I was an easy target. The exchange of money and the artifact was completed quickly. I was pleased with my bargaining tactics, and the boys had money in their pockets, probably to spend on sweets at the Hudson's Bay store.

After our noon meal, Chief Steward Moreau informed us that the water main had been turned off for repairs, which would take a few hours. We had to postpone cleaning the cabins.

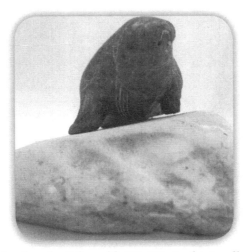

*Carving done by Eeloopalik #E5-746. Author's collection.*

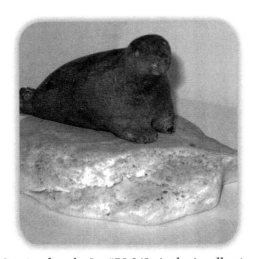

*Carving done by Joe #E5-848. Author's collection.*

Bill and I went to Cabin B-10 and shut the door, so we would not be disturbed. For the next two hours, we discussed many of the issues raised the previous evening with Dr. Oschinsky. We knew we were in no position to make changes, but sought to seek a favourable resolution, or at least a compromise.

Leaving the cabin, we ran into the chief steward. By the quizzical look on his face, we knew he wondered where we had been and what we had been up to. "The water system has been repaired. Finish up your cabins," he announced.

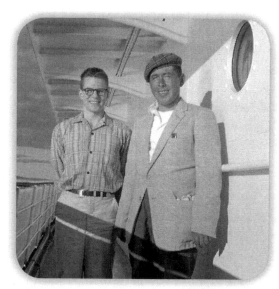

*The author and Tom on the Promenade Deck. Photo taken by Bill Kendall.*

Bill and I worked in tandem. Two to a cabin made quick work, and we managed to complete all our assigned cabins before the evening meal.

After dinner, I went out onto the Promenade Deck. There I met a man dressed in a sports jacket and wearing a tartan tam. Shortly after we introduced ourselves, I asked him about his hat. Soon we were in deep discussion relating our personal histories. Tom was thirty-three years old, he spoke Eskimo and English, and he was employed by the Hudson's Bay store. His mother was an Eskimo and his father was a whaler from Scotland. The hospitable nature of the Eskimos kept his father and other whalers safe, warm, and well fed throughout the long winter. It was a delightful and informative conversation, and we parted friends.

With the medical survey for this settlement completed, the barges and surf boats were secured to the decks. Soon after, we weighed anchor and said goodbye to this beautiful settlement. Our next destination: Eric Cove and the settlement of Ivujivik, the northernmost settlement in Quebec.

We arrived at Eric Cove around eleven in the morning. It was a beautiful sight, despite the foggy conditions, with high hills on either side and a small valley at the base of the cove. The small settlement of Ivujivik seemed to be nestled in the valley hugging

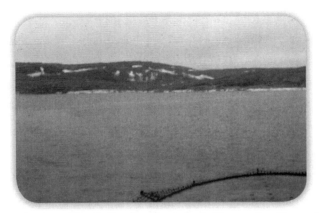

*Settlement of Ivujivik taken from the helicopter landing pad.
Author's collection.*

the coastline. This was our second visit; we had been here before our first stop at Cape Dorset.

As the CGS *N.B. McLean* was anchored in the cove, we were able to transfer mail before pushing off to our next destination, Port Harrison.[5]

Every day, usually after the evening meal, I would return to my cabin to take advantage of some quiet time for writing in my diary about the day's events. Some of the information I obtained from the hydrographers' office, some from notices posted on board, and some from just listening and being involved.

It was cool and overcast, and the *Howe*'s forward progress was at half speed. The ice in Hudson Bay and the foggy conditions slowed the ship. The ice reconnaissance report from the helicopter pilot stated there was heavy pack ice for a radius of thirty miles around the ship. This meant a further reduction in speed as the quartermaster sought out various safe courses.

I saw a notice of sale for an Eskimo parka (Grenfell cloth outer shell and wool inner shell with wolf fur surrounding the hood), which I purchased for $30. It fit me well. It had been sewn by an Eskimo woman on board, and I considered it a special keepsake of this northern tour. The more I came in contact with the Eskimos on board, the more I came to appreciate the work put into the making of their clothing. Every item, from head to toe, was made largely from seals, a staple for both food and clothing. For their

---

5   Inukjuak, Quebec.

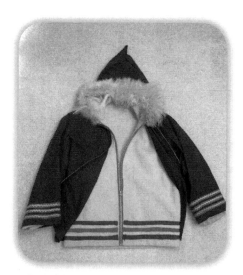

*Eskimo parka purchased by author, which was donated to the Museum of Civilization in July 2011. Author's collection.*

mukluks, the women would spend long hours chewing the sealskin before forming it into boots suitable for prolonged outdoor wear; any stitching was done with sinew. Arduous work, but the results speak for themselves.

On the evening of Saturday, July 18, the Executive Suite hosted the following: Officer-in-Charge / Eastern Arctic Patrol, Dr. Stevens; Drs. Ruth McLeesh, R.M. Lane, and Oschinsky; nurse Madeline Onslow; student technician Cort Beckingham; and Alex, an interpreter for Dr. Oschinsky. Dr. Oschinsky kept us laughing with his tales of "six-legged crud" (a figment of his imagination), and soon others were adding their own embellishments. Laughter filled the Suite, providing a welcome change from the tense atmosphere that had come to characterize the ship.

How did this soiree come about in the light of restrictions ordered down from the Bridge? I assume that the passengers, although fully informed, didn't care. In the end, it was a fun evening, a most pleasant get-together enjoyed by all.

We arrived in Port Harrison in the early hours of Sunday morning, July 19. The *Howe* anchored a couple of miles from shore, and I went out onto the Promenade Deck to see this port of call. Several buildings hugged the shoreline, and I concluded this was one of the better developed communities we had visited. I could make out from the deck a mission house, the Hudson's Bay Company store, an RCMP post, and a Department of Transport station. This was also the settlement from which Eskimo families and their possessions were transported on board the *Howe* and moved to Grise Fiord and Resolute Bay in 1953.

We were reassigned our cabin responsibilities, again, and I was assigned Dr. Oschinsky's cabin. While a change is as good as a rest, I suppose, I was uncertain as to whether this change was for the better. The good doctor was known as "Seven Blankets" Oschinsky, due to his habit of sleeping under that many blankets. Making up his bed, therefore, was a real chore, made even more difficult when the linen had to be changed.

Quartermaster Barbeau joined us in our cabin for a visit after dinner, which he didn't do nearly so often as before. Had someone spoken to him, too? Was he on a directed mission? In the past, we had learned much about the ship's inner workings and heard stories of northern adventures. On this occasion, he spoke openly about significant events on board, which made us think that maybe he was trying to gain our confidence. Was he looking to get information out of us in exchange? In the end, I doubt it.

After Mr. Barbeau left the cabin, I went up on deck. There was a full moon, and the ripples on the water fascinated me, causing my thoughts to drift. I recalled other moonlit nights at the cottage. It was one of those precious moments to be cherished forever: Nature showcasing her beauty in a picture-perfect setting.

We weighed anchor and set course across Hudson Bay for Churchill, Manitoba.

Besides doing our chores, we were required to polish the ship's brass fittings. This was a big job, and Chief Steward Moreau kept a close eye on our work. Some items were badly tarnished, meaning they had to be re-polished up to three times. The ship had to be in first-class shape upon arrival in Churchill. Were we expecting special visitors there?

It was going on eleven o'clock in the evening, and we were in our cabin reading and chatting quietly when a loud knock sounded on our door, causing us to jump to attention. There was Chief Steward Moreau. "This is an inspection!" he announced. Standing behind him were stewards Leaping Louis and The Bass. Was this the Enforcers Committee? There was a party going on two decks above us, which we could clearly hear in our cabin, deep in the bowels of the ship.

They stated there were rumours we had broken the captain's restrictions for fraternizing and that the captain suspected we were at the party. Too bad! Disappointment showed clearly on the faces of the chief and his sidekicks. They would have to inform the captain that all was well below decks.

We had a good chuckle over this. However, an undercurrent of suspicion, tension, and low morale continued to permeate the ship, and it was obvious that the senior officers were anxious to catch us in violation of orders. If successful, they could then discharge us at Churchill, where we could easily obtain transportation south. It would be a simple and convenient solution.

Tuesday, July 21, dawned bright and sunny—a good day for sailing. We proceeded to make up cabins, but we were delayed as many passengers were still asleep. We were not sorry to have missed the party; in fact, it had given us an opportunity to gloat amongst ourselves. We had put a dilly over on the "Weasel"—the captain—who tried to catch us doing the naughty. When might the Enforcers Committee strike again? While these events seem trivial, they illustrated just how low morale had become. We knew the officers viewed us with skepticism, but were they looking for transgression worthy of throwing us in the brig? (Yes, there was one on board, according to Quartermaster Barbeau.) Or at least ordered off the ship at Churchill?

I had a most interesting chat with Robbie Levack, the helicopter pilot, that afternoon in his cabin. Robbie had spent several years flying in the North and had many fascinating stories to tell.

On most occasions, Robbie wore his flying gear: an over-jacket with a large pouch in front and a badge on the left sleeve with Resolute Bay emblazoned across the top; an officer's peaked cap with a black band and gold insignia; and sunglasses. He looked just like he'd just completed a sortie over Europe from the last war.

I asked him about some of the items he had on display in his cabin.

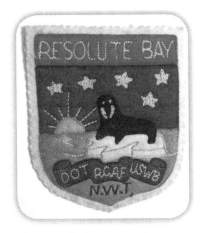

*Resolute Bay Badge. Author's collection.*

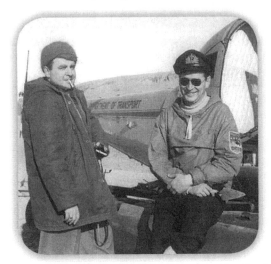

*Robbie on helicopter with Dr. O. Photo courtesy of Dr. Ruth McLeese.*

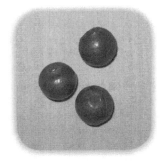

*Grapeshot. Author's collection.*

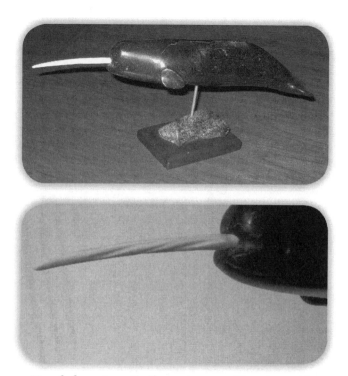

*Narwhal carvings. Artifacts courtesy of Lyn Arsenault.*

"On previous trips into the North," he began, "I landed on peaks not covered in ice. At my feet, there would be all these fossils scattered about. I just scooped them up and brought them back to the ship." He placed a couple of items in my hand.

"They look as though they might have been sea creatures. Do you know anything else about them?" I asked.

"No, sorry. I collected them in hopes that I would find someone who could tell me something about them. I guess when we get back south, I will try to learn more."

I was curious as to the origin of a piece of ivory about three feet long, lying on the floor of his cabin, almost under his bed. It was a front tooth from a narwhal. It was quite heavy, and I noticed it looked like a screw, with ridges spiralling down its length. Robbie told me that the narwhal lives in the Arctic and was a staple of the Eskimo diet. The Eskimos used this "tooth" to carve sculptures as well as walking sticks. Due to its rarity, it could also fetch a handsome price in the south.

Short, staccato knocks sounded on the cabin door, and the captain popped his head into Robbie's cabin. He glanced quickly around, his eyes focusing on me. He scowled, made a few general comments, then he praised Robbie for his flying skills in retrieving the patient from Resolution Island in dangerous weather conditions. Several days had passed since then. Was the Weasel checking up on me? Was this considered fraternizing with the passengers?

That afternoon, our chores included washing and waxing the dining salon and the companionways. The *C.D. Howe* was ready as best we could make her for our arrival in Churchill—and whatever might transpire there.

# Chapter Six

# The Port of Churchill, Hudson Bay

The port of Churchill was the gateway for shipping wheat and other commodities from the prairie provinces to overseas markets. I, therefore, assumed it would be a large port with a number of quays to handle many ocean-going vessels at one time, and I looked forward to our arrival. After being at sea for four weeks, we would have an opportunity to leave the ship's confines, widen our horizons, and explore the town, the site of which had been a settlement and gathering place for centuries.

Arriving at Churchill had other implications, as well. Would we, the cabin stewards, carry out our threat to phone Ottawa with our complaints or leave the ship? Would the senior officers, along with the head of the medical team, collaborate and provide Ottawa with a half-time report? We expected some sort of change to happen, but there were still more questions than answers.

In the meantime, the ship circled in the waters off Churchill awaiting arrival of the pilot, who, upon taking command, would manoeuvre the *Howe* safely up the Churchill River to her assigned berth.

I finished making up my cabins, then stepped out on deck to watch the seamen handle the heavy lines and moor the ship. Thick lines both fore and aft were tossed ashore and looped over the bollards alongside the concrete pier. Spring lines, both fore and aft, were fastened to the bollards to offset the forward and backward movement of the ship caused by the river's current and the rising and falling tide. The gangplank was lowered and secured. From the Bridge, the captain and ship's officers issued orders to the seamen below, both on board and on the pier, as they adjusted the lines until the captain was satisfied the ship was secured.

The port was much smaller and with fewer quays than I had anticipated. There were, however, railway tracks alongside the quays to facilitate movement of grain and other commodities from the freight cars to the ocean freighters. It all appeared well organized. Two ships were moored alongside the quays: the CGS *C.D. Howe* and the CGS *N.B. McLean*.

After lunch, I left the ship and walked back along the quay to the *McLean*. One of my school friends and a neighbour in Ottawa, Mike Harris, was a crew member on this ship. Mike stood about a head taller than me and, together, we looked like the popular comic characters, Mutt and Jeff.

We met up and shared stories of our adventures to date. Mike shared his cabin with one other seaman, which was posh compared to mine. It appeared quite homey—a comfortable refuge at the end of a busy day.

Mike gave me a quick lesson on the *McLean*. "This ship is a veteran ice-breaker. It is shorter in length than the *Howe* [260 feet versus 295 feet] and has a top speed of about fifteen knots. The engine capacity is substantial: the four boilers provide lots of power to tackle any ice conditions," he explained.

It was a more powerful ship than the *Howe*; a true work horse, I thought.

"The *McLean* has the power to ride up on the ice floes and break the ice creating safe passage for other ships," Mike continued. "It is not as new a ship as the *Howe*, as it's been in service since the 1930s; you can see evidence of the ship's age. But she is a solid, seaworthy ship. I'm enjoying working with the officers and crew."

I told Mike about the various jobs assigned to me thus far in the voyage, the medical emergency on Resolution Island, and the difficulties traversing the strait under severe weather and ice conditions. I wondered if our paths would cross again during the patrol.

"I am not sure at this point," replied Mike, "although we have sailed pretty much in tandem over the past few weeks. We are scheduled to go to Resolute Bay in a few weeks. Who knows, maybe we will meet again."

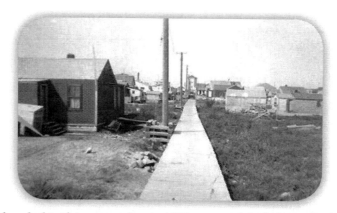

*Although this photo was taken in 1956, not much had changed when I visited three years later. This area was known as the Boardwalk, because of the box built to cover a steam-heated waterline, believed to have been constructed to supply the Roman Catholic mission seen at the far end. Any of the residences along the Boardwalk were allowed to install water taps for their own use. Photo by Doug Stewart.*

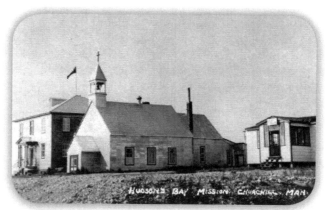

*Town hall, mission, and museum, Churchill, Manitoba. Photo by Ed Smith.*

What a welcome change to enjoy the company of and share stories and experiences with a good friend from home, so far away from home.

Bill and I signed out later in the afternoon to tour downtown Churchill. This was the first time we had set foot on *terra firma* since Quebec. However, the two places could not have been more different. At the end of the concrete pier was a road, which was more of a dirt track. Ruts with tall grass growing in the middle provided evidence of some vehicular traffic, but not much. It looked more like a farm lane in the south than a major road to town.

Down the road, we walked past a cluster of narrow, single-storey, grey and white wooden houses. They all looked like they were built from the same plan. We got a quick glimpse of the inside of one, when a mother opened the door to let out a pet and call the children in. It was, in our minds, rudimentary housing, but adequate.

We visited the Eskimo Museum and the Hudson's Bay store. The former was thought-provoking. Although it did not have a large collection, it provided an overview of the settlement's history. In addition to the artifacts, there were pictures of Churchill landmarks. We noticed that there were few amenities for leisure activities. Perhaps those who lived here were too busy attending to life's necessities to have much time for leisure, or to worry about entertaining those passing through, like us.

The dusty main street featured a few businesses fronted by a wooden boardwalk; it was reminiscent of main streets seen on old westerns. It was apparent that these buildings, as well as the schools and churches, were erected in a hodge-podge arrangement with no attention to town planning.

That evening, Bill and I joined up with some fellows from the *McLean* and went into town to the "Igloo," to see *A Night to Remember*, starring Kenneth More. This 1958 movie featured the tragic sinking of the RMS *Titanic* half a century before. Many of the images struck a little too close to home. What if something similar would happen to us? We had experienced situations in which heavy ice packs not only impeded the *Howe*'s progress, but caused the ship to shudder and stop.

After the movie, we went to the bowling lanes to catch the action and perhaps play a few games. However, all the lanes were taken, so we went to the local restaurant, which was full of customers, too. With little else to amuse ourselves, we decided to return to our respective ships. Despite finding little to do, we shared adventures, told jokes, and had some laughs. In all, it was a memorable evening.

To top it off, we received a large quantity of mail from family and friends. The news from home was welcome, indeed. Although I had written many letters to family and friends since leaving Quebec, they had not reached their destination before these incoming letters had been written. Answers to any questions I had asked would have to wait until the next mail. While frustrating, it encouraged me to write more letters.

The next day, Chief Steward Moreau gave us extra duties, polishing the interior passageways and equipment; it was all part of making a good impression for our important, albeit mysterious, guests. All companionways, stairs, and passages were washed and waxed to a high shine.

It was a beautiful, sunny, and warm day. By noon, I had completed my duties, so I decided to do more sightseeing and set out to explore on my own. I took my time examining the structure of the buildings and thinking about the inhabitants' way of life here. I walked past a small schoolhouse, which was closed for the summer; the neighbouring playing field was overgrown with grass. I wandered around the cemetery, reading the names and dates inscribed on the markers. These marked the graves of those whose legacy was the life and times of this settlement.

After the evening meal in the mess, our special guest arrived: the Deputy Minister of Northern Affairs and National Resources. I was introduced to him, as were other members of the crew. I hoped he and his companions noticed the results of our hard work and were pleased with the *Howe*'s shipshape condition.

On our last full day in Churchill, the sky was overcast and the temperature cooler. Final preparations were under way, and we worked longer than normal. The seamen, with our assistance, loaded cargo and supplies for the next leg of the voyage.

In addition to taking on more cargo and fuel, the *Howe* also had taken on more passengers and Eskimos. There was no mention of, or any decision on, however, the earlier troubles. I assumed our talks with some of the passengers had had a positive effect. It appeared, on the surface anyway, that all was well, at least for the time being.

July 25. Departure Day. It had rained most of the night leaving puddles all over the pier.

The day before, I had tried to place a long distance call to my girlfriend in Ottawa; however, the operator told me that there were no available lines out of Churchill. I would have to try again when the lines were not as busy. At 7 a.m., I signed off, figuring this was my last chance to make that phone call. I ran to the payphone located on the quay and hoped that the lines would not be busy at this early hour. I dialled through the operator and requested a long distance collect call to Liz's home. Her father answered the phone.

"Hello."

"May I speak to Liz? It's Murray. I am calling from Churchill, Manitoba." Fortunately, he recognized my voice and did not scold me for phoning so early. It was 8 a.m. in Ottawa.

"Just a minute, I'll see if she is up."

Although it was only a few minutes until Liz came to the phone, it seemed much longer. When I heard Liz's voice, I was overjoyed. It was so good to hear her and I felt as if she were close by. I apologized for the early call, but the ship was preparing to leave port. I had many questions to ask, but the operator came on the line to inform me that my three minutes were up. Although our call was short, it was still heartwarming to hear a familiar voice from home.

While walking back to the ship, I pondered the contents of our conversation and felt empty. Had I made a mistake making this call, or was it realizing the great distance between us? The voyage was only about half over. I would be at sea for another two months. With a sigh, I tucked these thoughts away. It was time for breakfast and to get back to work.

One of the crew from the hydrographic team, Dave Simpson, disembarked at Churchill shortly before we sailed, so as to return home. I knew him from Ottawa. We had spent winter weekends racing at the Camp Fortune ski hill.

We had been in port for three days.

The sky was overcast as we pulled away from our mooring at 8:45 a.m. Shortly thereafter, we left the harbour and dropped the pilot. There was a light drizzle falling and a strong wind blowing. Leaving the Churchill River and entering Hudson Bay, the ship took on its distinctive rock and roll. I thought I had sea legs, now, but this was going to be a good test. As the port of Churchill slipped behind us in the mist, I realized the next time we moored to a pier would be in Quebec City, at the conclusion of the voyage; a sobering thought.

# Chapter Seven

# On to the Arctic Circle

A s Churchill faded in the distance, I looked back at this small landfall. I had enjoyed our short stay. During shore leave, I had a chance to explore the small town, make some new acquaintances, and talk to my girlfriend back home. I was also feeling homesick. Perhaps it was because we were now on the second half of our journey, but we still had many miles of sea to traverse and numerous settlements to visit.

Enough of this moping! There was work to be done, and I thought it best to get right at it. That would distract me from my thoughts. However, I soon realized that accomplishing my tasks was going to take longer than anticipated. There had been several parties on board the previous evening, and many of the passengers were still asleep. I couldn't get into a number of cabins to make them up.

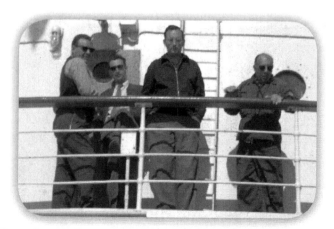

*From L to R: Dr. L. Oschinsky, Dr. A.H. Stevens, Dr. R.M. Lane, and Dr. Smithurst. Author's collection.*

It was a beautiful, sunny day. The Bay was calm, and the sun bounced off the water, making millions of sparkling diamonds. Slowly, the passengers appeared, a little groggy, to soak up the sun.

I grabbed my camera and headed up to the helicopter deck, where I captured this picture of the doctors on the Boat Deck enjoying the fine weather.

We were headed for Southampton Island and the settlement of Coral Harbour, then on to Nottingham Island. I wondered where these names originated and who was responsible for so naming them. I recalled the chat I had with Tom at Cape Dorset, whose father was a whaler from Scotland. Did the whalers from earlier expeditions name these settlements to honour familiar places back home?

Dr. Oschinsky was a noted physical anthropologist at the Department of Anthropology, Victoria Museum, in Ottawa. He had a personality quite unlike anyone else I knew; a smiling demeanour, yet a no-nonsense approach regarding matters of a more serious nature. He was well liked among his colleagues. He also spent time visiting us in our cabin, paying little regard for the edict prohibiting this activity. He often shared humorous stories, as well as offered up sage advice.

During this voyage into the Eastern Arctic, Dr. Oschinsky was conducting individual surveys of the Eskimos. He measured and recorded their physical characteristics, such as their height and weight, facial features, and dental configurations.

Shortly after I had snapped the picture of the doctors on the Boat Deck, Dr. Oschinsky approached me.

"I need an assistant to record my research findings, and I am prepared to pay you for your time. Your assistance would be appreciated."

After confirming my interest in accepting his offer, Dr. Oschinsky agreed to speak to Chief Steward Moreau and arrange my secondment.

The next day, I arrived at his little office, where I saw, in addition to a table and chairs, a weigh scale and an assortment of instruments. I was baffled. With the exception of the weigh scale, I did not recognize any of the pieces of equipment. The doctor, however, proved to be a good teacher.

"Many Eskimos today exhibit traces of Caucasian physical characteristics," he said to me as I sat on a stool with several papers on the table before me. "I hope this research may uncover some examples of the Eskimos' original racial characteristics. This may be akin to looking for a needle in a haystack.

"You must put the name and Eskimo number of the individual and the name of the settlement at the top," he instructed. "I will take the measurements, and then relate the information to you for recording." This was an opportunity for me to learn more about our northern neighbours. I agreed to assist him as best I could and showed my eagerness to get the job done accurately.

We dropped anchor at Coral Harbour early in the morning of July 27. I was struck as to how small the settlement was. From the deck, all I could see were a few buildings and tents hugging the shoreline. I later discovered there was an air strip that had been built during the war. As in other communities, Eskimos gathered along the shore to greet the *Howe*. Shortly after the anchor was set, the medical survey began and there was a lot of hustle and bustle as the Eskimos were transported to and from the ship.

Dr. Oschinsky, with me as his assistant, began the anthropological survey after the Eskimos had completed their medicals. Our clients did not exhibit any fear; in fact, they were curious as to what we were doing. There was lots of loud laughter, pointing of fingers at others, and, of course, their high-pitched voices as they chided each other and chatted amongst themselves. I was kept busy recording the data as Dr. Oschinsky rhymed it off.

Dr. Oschinsky had a special mould filled with a pliable substance into which he asked the Eskimos to "Take a bite." This prompted more laughter as they thought the doctor was giving them something to eat. Their sour expressions said otherwise. Later, plaster of Paris would be prepared and poured into the mould. When this casting dried, the doctor would have an imprint of the Eskimo's teeth, which would be used for further study.

The approximately 150 Eskimos who came through the medical/dental survey were a hardy group of individuals. Dr.

Smithurst, the dentist, told me later that he had done ten extractions and sixteen fillings.

"Why so many?" I asked. I assumed their diet of nature's bounty would not give rise to decayed teeth.

"You may be correct," he stated, "but many Eskimos buy sweets at the Hudson's Bay store. Extractions, in lieu of fillings, are quick. We make brief visits to the settlements, so there is no opportunity for a followup."

In addition to the sweets, I also assumed that it was not common practice amongst the Eskimo to brush their teeth.

I subsequently discovered that these settlements were cashless. While people had incomes, obtained by trading furs and other goods or receiving government pensions, there were no coins or bank notes. When an individual would go into a Hudson's Bay store to purchase goods, the value would be subtracted from their allowance and recorded on a chit. A rather sensible system, as I do not recall any Eskimo who had a pocket sewn into their pants, or carried a wallet or a purse.

As Dr. Oschinsky and I continued with the survey, I noted that many of the Eskimos could speak some English. Unfortunately, not many southerners had learned their language. While Dr. Oschinsky had an interpreter, Alex, he did not need to use his services often.

One man who came to us for measurement stated that he been born in 1886, making him seventy-three years old. Although he had passed his medical and was in fine spirits, not many Eskimo reached such an advanced age, as their society could not support individuals who could not pull their weight. It was a known fact that when an elder became incapacitated, a younger member would remove that person from the family. Fortunately, with the advent of pensions, the older generation could still contribute to the family, even though they may no longer be able to hunt and fish.

Before we completed our work for the day, Dr. Oschinsky asked that I give him an impression of my teeth. "Why?" I asked. He explained that the predominant "shovel-shaped" front teeth of the Caucasian differed from the Eskimo, whose front teeth either had a small degree of "shovel-shape," or none at all. This would be a key to determining the extent that Caucasian racial traits appeared amongst the Eskimo. These traits were a result of liaisons with Europeans, like Tom, whose father had been a whaler from Scotland.

The doctor would use my dental mould as a comparison in his anthropological findings of the Eskimos. This evidence would be the basis of a research paper he would later write and present.

One man we met had two wives. He referred to them as his senior wife and junior wife. It was not clear as to the circumstances behind this, but it was not surprising. If a man dies, it was the accepted practice for the widow (and her children) to join up with another provider. Survival is a strong instinct. Thus, a logical arrangement was to become a second wife.

Shortly thereafter, I met a man who, although only twenty years old, was married and had children. He was only a year older than me. I thought being a family man at that age was a big step, but taking into consideration the harsh environment in which they lived, it was understandable why early marriages were the norm, rather than the exception.

There was a DEW (Distant Early Warning) Line airstrip at Coral Harbour. Wheeler Airlines would fly out Eskimos diagnosed with tuberculosis to sanitariums, either in Montreal or Hamilton, for medical care. The plane would also take outgoing mail from the ship.

For a couple of days, I had been very ill. I suffered from severe abdominal pains and could not keep any food down. I tried to keep up with my responsibilities, but my cabin mate, Bill, was forced to fill in where he could. We got the job done, but barely. By Wednesday, three days into the ordeal, I was not functioning at all. I was tired and the pains were unbearable. In my mind, I could not care less what happened next.

Dr. Ruth McLeese, the ship's chief medical officer, came to the cabin to assess my condition. She commented that I must have picked up a bug from something I had eaten. I had never been this ill before. Dr. McLeese gave me some medication. Later, I discovered there were others with similar symptoms.

I now divided my time between running to the head and sleeping. I had little concern for anything other than surviving and getting better soon.

I was told the weather was poor with heavy clouds and stiff winds to rock the ship, but I knew I was not seasick. This felt much different than the motion sickness endured at the beginning of the trip, although any thought of food would prompt the regurgitation reflex. Oops, here we go again!

Poor weather conditions hindered progress and increased the travel time from Coral Harbour. The *Howe* finally dropped anchor at Nottingham Island at 3 a.m. on July 30. The helicopter began ferrying Eskimos for their medical examinations, and the crew began unloading cargo. The medical survey and the cargo work were completed by 6 a.m. The anchor was then raised and we set sail for Cape Dorset, just as we were roused for breakfast and the start of our daily chores.

Many of the medical and support staff in turn went to their cabins to grab a few hours of sleep, meaning we could not complete our duties. We, therefore, returned to our cabin to rest and read until lunch.

At 7 p.m., we dropped anchor at Cape Dorset. The crew began unloading cargo taken on at Churchill for the Northern Affairs and National Resources representative. In addition, more than a hundred Eskimos had returned to Dorset from their summer camp; they were required to go through the medical survey.

At 7:30 p.m., Dr. Oschinsky, with me as his assistant, commenced the survey. Our work continued past midnight.

With the cargo unloaded and the medical survey finished, the *Howe* weighed anchor for Lake Harbour.

As this was a sailing day, the passengers and crew could relax somewhat. The early risings of the past few mornings to conduct the medical survey and unload cargo meant that everyone needed a breather.

It was the last day in July; summer was half over. It did not look much like summer, though. The sky was dull, with heavy grey clouds. Occasionally hints of sun would break through, but the temperature remained a cool 60°F.

The helicopter pilot, Robbie, and a nurse, Faith, were playing with a one-month-old husky pup. The pup was quite energetic and enjoyed the activity. I liked dogs, and had fun playing with the pup, too. I thought it would be great to bring a pup home at the conclusion of the trip.

"You best give this more thought," Robbie replied.

Faith agreed. "You may have fun with the pup now, but how are you going to feed him? You have to have a place to keep him on board while you are working."

They emphasized that the pup was "adjusted to the North" and that he might have difficulty acclimatizing to life in the south. I reluctantly agreed with them, and in retrospect, cooler minds prevailed.

As the settlement of Lake Harbour slowly disappeared from view, it was difficult to believe we had spent so little time at this port of call. Not only was the medical survey completed, but Dr. Oschinsky had completed his anthropological recordings of Eskimos.

I finished my work for Dr. Oschinsky in time for a surprise visit from Rick Clark, a friend from Ottawa. Rick had come over from the CGS *Edward Cornwallis*, which was anchored across the bay.

Rick and I had been classmates through elementary and secondary school. We shared a passion for skiing and had inaugurated a high school ski team, much to the principal's displeasure, who viewed this sport as being injury-prone. He had previously resisted any ventures to start a ski team under the school's name, but when the team placed well in several competitions, he seemed to have a change of heart.

Our visit was brief, but still time enough to compare shipboard experiences and get caught up on the news from home and other relevant events happening elsewhere. Too soon it was time for Rick to return to his ship. They were slated to go on to Churchill.

On this day, the weather was bright, sunny, and warm, with a slight breeze, similar to the day before. I took several trips around the deck. It was an occasion not only to enjoy the fine weather, but to see the distant shoreline; it was beautiful in the northern sense, rocky and grey, with small patches of vegetation. This pleasant weather did not happen often, so it was a bonus to have both a picturesque view and the time to enjoy it.

There was another change in cabin assignments. I gave up one of my cabins for the dubious distinction of being assigned to the wireless radio officer's cabin. I was advised by my cabin mates that Mr. Laxton was known as a stickler for detail, who considered cleanliness and neatness a high priority, and would voice his complaints if not satisfied. This cabin was located on the Bridge Deck; one of the larger cabins, it had a bed-sitting room and a separate washroom.

I was now faced with a daunting responsibility. If the job was not done to his satisfaction, the officer was inclined to complain to the chief steward about the shoddy work and demand his cabin be re-done. I assumed, quite rightly as it turned out, that I needed to ensure his cabin was spotless and make his bed to military standards. To add to the challenge, there was no interior access to this cabin. I had to haul my cleaning tools, pails, mops, and rags, up an exterior ladder, which was perpendicular to the deck leading to the Bridge Deck. I pictured myself hanging on for dear life, equipment dangling from arms and legs, as the ship ploughed up and down through rough seas, before I even began making up the cabin.

I did not fear heights, but the fact of the matter was that the Bridge Deck was the topmost deck, two decks above the Promenade Deck. While the view from this vantage point was amazing, in rough seas, the rolling of the ship would be unnerving.

It was a bit scary, the first few times I ascended the ladder to access Mr. Laxton's cabin. "Do not look down" was my mantra. Fortunately, I soon overcame my trepidation of climbing a ladder at a ninety-degree angle, allowing me to focus my attention on the real job at hand.

We left Hudson Strait, sailing around Resolution Island, and headed northward through Davis Strait along the coast of Baffin Island. We skirted the leading edge of a large ice pack and sighted many growlers and icebergs. I saw one that resembled a schooner. It was a very pretty sight. Our noon position was in close proximity to the CGS *Montcalm* and mail was transferred to this ship by helicopter.

Usually, after our noon meal, we would return to our cabin for some quiet time. On this occasion, Bill asked me if I knew how to

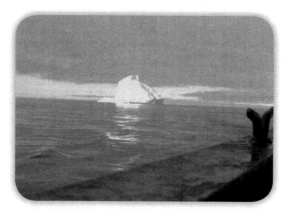

*Iceberg off the coast of Baffin Island. Author's collection.*

play cribbage. I recalled that my grandfather played this card game, but I did not know how. Bill said he would teach me, and if the other cabin boys knew how to play, we could have tournaments.

I quickly picked up the rules, and cribbage became a regular feature of our noon-hour period of relaxation. If one walked by our cabin door, one would hear shouts of "15-2, 15-4," and so on as the points were tallied. I, oftentimes, ended up with low scores. Regardless, it was an enjoyable way to pass the time.

Approaching the end of the sixth week, we sailed into Lancaster Sound. There were increased incidents of ice in the form of growlers, heavy pack ice, and large, beautifully sculpted icebergs of brilliant colours. The sea was almost completely covered with some type of ice formation. We would soon be crossing the Arctic Circle, 66° 33′ N Lat., another milestone in this adventure.

# Chapter Eight

# Crossing the Arctic Circle, Davis Strait

W e proceeded making our way northward in Baffin Bay towards Lancaster Sound. The ship was sailing into a strong headwind, which set the ship tossing in the waves. I did not experience any feelings of illness, so could now say with full confidence that I had my sea legs. The days progressed with little change in the daily routine and no major issues. Yet, once again, the ship travelled at reduced speed due to foggy conditions as well as scattered ice.

At 6 a.m., Tuesday, August 4, the *Howe* crossed the Arctic Circle.

The news of a celebration in honour of Crossing the Circle spread throughout the ship. A few individuals had already approached me, asking if I had ever crossed the Arctic Circle before, and when I replied that I had not, they indicated that I was a likely candidate for an initiation ceremony, where I would be presented to King Neptune. I conjured up indignities that I and other initiates on board might be subjected to; someone suggested an impromptu performance of one's thespian talents. Since there were a number who would be initiated, the ceremony promised to be an entertaining event.

Just before our evening meal, we were in our cabin when we heard a couple of light knocks on our door. As I opened the door, towering before me stood the first mate. I immediately thought, what had we done now? Although previous edicts and restrictions had seemingly been relaxed, or at least ignored, you can well imagine my concern.

He smiled. "You are invited to attend the Circle Crossing Party this evening in the salon," he said. "This special occasion is for everyone, but specifically for those for whom this is their first time crossing the Arctic Circle. You will be inaugurated into the Loyal Order of Circle Crossers, under the rule of King Neptune." A collective sigh of relief from all cabin boys echoed round the cabin. It was an invitation, rather than an interrogation and reprimand.

"On occasions such as this, you are required to wear a white shirt and be dressed appropriately for presentation to the king."

"Why a white shirt?" I asked. Was a white shirt regulation for special ceremonies?

"A good white shirt, not your work tunic. Do the best you can," said the first mate, then he briefly outlined the format of the party and the procedures for the ceremony. It sounded as though this was a party for everyone on board. We wondered if past indiscretions were bygones. Only time would tell.

We accepted the invitation with thanks, and with that, the first mate left the cabin.

As we sat down to discuss what we could do as a performance, we felt that a few drams of Highland Heather were needed to fortify us for the forthcoming indignities. Bill and Sandy suggested a rousing verse of the Queen's University football song, "Oil thigh na Banrighinn." Both Bill and Sandy were first year students at Queen's. Although the words were in Gaelic, the tune was simple, and we could flub the lines safely believing that none in the audience would be the wiser. Sandy and Bill gave a demonstration, then we practised a few times before declaring ourselves ready for the festivities.

Upon arrival in the main salon of the ship, we were greeted by the entire medical staff, the ship's officers of the Bridge, including the captain, the night waiter (whom we barely knew, as our paths rarely crossed), plus other staff and crew.

As instructed, Bill and I walked into the salon, followed by Sandy and Bob. The assembled guests turned and looked at us, sizing us up. While I recognized a few, I immediately felt out of place. What if I made a misstep, some social faux pas? I feared that I would humiliate myself, not only because we were in the spotlight, but because of my perceived negative standing in the captain's eyes.

At one end of the salon, I saw trays of finger food and light snacks on display, that were both pleasing to the eye as well as to the palate, as I soon discovered. The galley staff had gone to great lengths to serve up their best for this special party. We took our plates and filled them with goodies. We also helped ourselves to punch served in a large urn, which we quickly discovered had been liberally spiked with alcool. It was rumoured that overindulgence might result in unfavourable outcomes.

"Hear ye, hear ye," we heard the master of ceremonies announce over a small PA system. "The initiation 'pageant' is about to begin. King Neptune has arrived. All subjects must get down on one knee and recognize this exalted personage." Amidst laughter, I caught a glimpse of King Neptune. Who was he? He had to be someone from on board, as no one had been flown in recently by helicopter.

The mythical King of the Sea sat on his throne, his trident dripping with seaweed. In a sonorous voice, King Neptune pronounced how we were to proceed, "You will come before me, genuflect, and get down on one knee. I will place my trident on your shoulder, and you will repeat the oath after me. You will then perform all edicts issued by me." He then gave a brief statement of the ceremony's history and significance.

The ceremony would be completed once the inductee had performed a special act as ordered by King Neptune before the assembled. "On successful completion of this order, you will be recognized as a loyal subject of mine," he declared.

So, one had to make an absolute fool of oneself before Neptune and his court. Those who came before us presented well-polished performances, which were received with loud and sustained applause by the audience.

It was now our turn. With an effort to overcome our bit of stage fright, we formed up in a line, centre stage. From our mouths and hearts we gave a rousing rendition of the Queen's University football song. We had no bagpipes, no kilts, and we couldn't hold a tune in a bucket, but with legs kicking high, like a Rockette at Radio City Music Hall, we sang:

*"Oil thigh na Banrighinn a'Banrighinn gu brath!*
*Oil thigh na Banrighinn a'Banrighinn gu brath!*
*Oil thigh na Banrighinn a'Banrighinn gu brath!*
*Cha-gheill! Cha-gheill! Cha-gheill!"*

When the laughter finally died down, King Neptune delivered his concluding remarks and then departed. The ceremony was

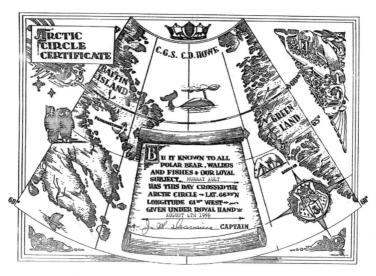

*Circle Crossing Certificate. Author's collection.*

over. All new members of Neptune's kingdom were presented with an official Circle Crossing Certificate, dated and signed by Captain J.M. Desrosiers.

The party continued for several hours, fuelled with good humour, high spirits, and even some dance music. While several couples took to the floor, I was at first hesitant to ask any of the ladies I knew there. Eventually, I asked Dr. McLeese for a dance and she accepted my invitation. It was a pleasant experience dancing to familiar tunes, and I felt accepted.

After the official party ended around 2 a.m., and people sought out various private parties that were springing up throughout the ship, Bill and I decided to go out on deck for a breath of fresh air.

"Who played the role of King Neptune?" I asked.

"I am not sure," he replied. "I thought it must have been an officer of the ship."

"I did, too. But as I looked around the salon, I didn't see anyone missing."

We were now in the "true" North, the Land of the Midnight Sun. It was light, as the sun did not set until 11:30 p.m., rising again at 2:30 a.m. I had brought my camera out on deck and took a picture of a large iceberg looming on the horizon with the first hints of sunrise glancing off it. It was three o'clock in the morning.

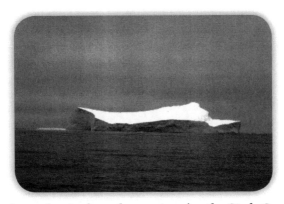

*Photo of iceberg taken in the early morning after the Circle Crossing Party.*
*Author's collection.*

The shape of the iceberg and the colours were amazing. I wanted a picture of this iceberg, not only to show family and friends back home, but as proof of the time of day and light available. I was pleased with the outcome of the final image.

Who was at the helm, I wondered. Was there a reliable lookout for icebergs? There must be several of the crew who were on the Bridge and in the engine room. I must have become so accustomed to the watch change bells that I no longer gave them any thought nor noticed them. Realization that the ship was under command twenty-four hours a day during the voyage was a given fact.

Come morning, there was nary a buzz on deck; the ship was very quiet. We attempted to make up a few cabins, but discovered many of the passengers were sound asleep, or did not want to be disturbed. We decided to put off doing our cabins until the afternoon, but still managed to complete them before dinner.

The partying also appeared to have affected the galley staff. The meals were on time, but they tasted awful. It was a sign of things to come.

As the days and weeks passed, the meals became more mundane and frequently had a freezer taste and smell. The chefs also seemed to have lost the imagination and will to create tasty dishes. For example, when hearing that bread pudding was on the menu for dessert, and that it was a culinary treat and favourite of French-Canadian kitchens, I decided to have a serving. It proved not a wise decision, as my taste buds reacted negatively after the first spoonful.

However, the chefs did manage to do themselves proud on the rare occasion. While bread pudding had been a disappointment, *pouding chômeur* was a treat! It consisted of white cake baked in a generous serving of maple syrup. I remembered my mother making this dessert, which she called cottage pudding. Regardless of its name, it was one of my favourites, and I and others had seconds. It brought to mind fond memories of home. On another occasion, the dessert menu featured maple sugar pie. No further comment needed. A French-Canadian dainty, whose reputation had spread into the Ottawa Valley.

It was a given that fish was the main entree on Fridays, in recognition of Roman Catholic practices at the time. For lunch and dinner, the menu featured two selections: one a specialty fish, such as baked cod; the other, usually salmon loaf. During the war years, I lived with my grandparents while my father served overseas, and my grandmother would often serve a delicious supper of salmon loaf. When it appeared on the Friday dinner menu on the ship, I placed my order for this in hopes that it would live up to my grandmother's version. I was not disappointed. It was grand! I ordered salmon loaf every Friday for the rest of the trip.

Except one Friday, when the menu featured fresh Arctic char. While I was familiar with the baked cod, this was new, and the seaman who waited for our orders was confronted with many questions.

"Where did this fish come from?" asked one of the seamen.

"What does it taste like?" I asked, as I was fairly picky about fish.

"How long has it been in the freezer?" asked Bill, my cabin mate.

The seaman replied, "I and a few of my friends caught this fish ourselves, and there is enough for everyone on board."

The seaman was proud of his success and gladly responded to the flood of questions. I went out on a limb and gave my order for what was later explained to me, a delicacy of the sea. With just one bite, I was overjoyed. This was a real delicacy. All too soon, my plate was empty. That exquisite taste of my first sampling of fresh Arctic char remains in my memory to this day.

Despite our grumblings, the chefs were to be commended.

Theirs was a task *extraordinaire*. They prepared nutritious meals under demanding conditions. There was no going out to the store for a special or missing ingredient. Regardless, they prepared three meals a day for everyone on board, as well as exceptional treats for special occasions, such as the Circle Crossing Party.

On this particular evening, we were privileged to enjoy a movie, *So This Is Paris*. Filmed in 1955, it starred Tony Curtis, Gloria DeHaven, and Gene Nelson. Most of the films we saw on board were old, almost vintage, featuring few if any Hollywood stars, and held little interest to me. This relatively recent musical comedy, however, was the perfect end to a delicious meal. The movies would also alternate between those with French and English dialogue. I remember seeing *Sabrina* (1954) starring Audrey Hepburn and Humphrey Bogart. The dialogue was dubbed in French, but I was able to follow and understand the storyline with little difficulty. I enjoyed it.

The next day, we returned to our regular schedule. While busy completing our tasks, Chief Steward Moreau conducted a snap inspection. Did he assume we were slacking off after the big party? He watched over us with eagle eyes as we carried out our cleaning tasks, but made no comments, either positive or negative. But we could tell by his expression what he thought. Perhaps this was a subtle warning that the edict still applied and the camaraderie experienced at the party was an exception to the rule.

That afternoon, I was asked to attend at the Medical Suite. The X-ray technician, Norm Harper, was attempting to take X-rays of three Eskimo babies, and he needed someone to hold them still. This was more difficult than it sounded. In the first place, the babies were accustomed to being held and gently cuddled by their mothers, a skill I did not have. I hung on firmly, fearing that I would drop the baby, which caused the baby to squirm. Vigorous yelling and even more squirming resulted when the baby realized that he was in a semi-dark room, with peculiar equipment, and in the arms of a stranger. Mr. Harper showed me how to hold the babies for optimum results, but the screaming only intensified. The parents tried to calm their children with soothing words, but to no avail. While the whole procedure took a relatively short time, I was very happy to return them to the welcoming arms of their parents. Miraculously, the crying and wailing stopped. What an experience!

Even though the day was sunny and bright, the temperature was cool, and for the past few hours, we had made limited progress due to the fog and the heavy ice conditions. Our revised destination was Arctic Bay. We became stuck in the ice for over two hours.

The ice prevented the *Howe* from getting close enough to drop anchor and carry out the mission at this post. The helicopter pilot conducted an ice reconnaissance flight and reported that Arctic Bay was packed solid with ice.

We could not see much of the settlement, due to billowy, white clouds hanging low to the ground. This was an unfamiliar sight to me, but perhaps common in the North.

We left Arctic Bay and returned to Lancaster Sound, but again fog and the floes of heavy packed ice made it impossible to proceed much above dead slow. Our next destination was Radstock Bay, but as ice hindered our progress, the ship dropped anchor to await better ice conditions.

The pace of activity on board matched the speed of the ship. On Saturday evening after dinner, we entertained Dr. Ruth McLeese in our cabin. It was a pleasant social visit, as we explored many topics of mutual interest.

Dr. McLeese had attended to me when I was ill with severe stomach pains a short while before. She had recently graduated from medical school at Dalhousie University in Halifax and was serving as the medical officer on board the CGS *C.D. Howe* for the Eastern Arctic Patrol. Although she had a no-nonsense approach, she was kind, gentle, and had a great deal of empathy, which I am sure she carried over to all her patients. I often thought she would make a good wife for some lucky guy.

Too soon the visit ended. Perhaps a hint of concern lingered regarding the edict against passengers visiting the Executive Suite. Hopefully, she would come again.

The next day proved the same as before, so the ship remained anchored. Later in the morning, Dr. Lane paid a house call to see Bill, who had a heavy cold and was most uncomfortable.

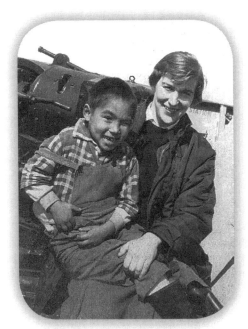

*Dr. Ruth McLeese. Author's collection.*

Accompanying him was Dr. McLeese, who wanted to take my blood pressure. It was normal, and I was left in a bit of a quandary as to why I merited the attention and why it took two doctors to carry out these simple tasks. Was there some concern as to the living conditions in the Executive Suite? Even though we did try to keep it as clean and livable as possible, there were limits as to what we could achieve.

The ship remained stuck in the ice for the third day. We were stuck in a rut, to say the least.

# Chapter Nine

# Resolute Bay, Cornwallis Island, Lancaster Sound

For five days, the *Howe* continued to steam slowly towards Resolute Bay. Each day slipped by with nary a significant event to distinguish it from the one before. As the *Howe* was only ice strengthened, the officers on the Bridge had to manoeuvre the ship through the ice to avoid damaging the hull, rather than break through. The ship's log indicated that the *Howe* was travelling at an average speed of 1.5 to 2 knots and progressed about fifty miles a day. The *Howe* had a mission to complete within a narrow window of time. The need to adhere to the scheduled visits to remote settlements on the one hand and deliver medical care and cargo to the inhabitants was jeopardized by the heavy ice conditions.

The menacing, heavy ice packs as far as the eye could see were a solemn reminder of the fate of the RMS *Titanic*.

The epic narrative poem, *The Titanic*, by E.J. Pratt, was required study in senior English courses when I was in high school. Born and raised in Newfoundland, Pratt's descriptions of icebergs were based on first-hand knowledge.

The poem opens at Harland and Wolff Works, Belfast, during the final stages in the building of this "unsinkable ship." The pride of the White Star Line, it was a marvel of engineering skill and elegant accoutrements, and was one of the largest, if not *the* largest and most luxurious ships to be built. It even included Marconi's state-of-the-art wireless communication link, which had been installed for safety purposes.

"She was fine when she left here!" exclaimed many a townie from Belfast who had witnessed the christening, which Pratt describes here:

> Glass crashed against the plates; a wine cascade,
> Netting the sunlight in a shower of pearls,
> Baptized the bow and gave the ship her name;
> . . .
> The perfect ship at last—the first unsinkable,
> Proved in advance—had not the folders read so?
> . . .
> And this belief had reached its climax when,
> Through wireless waves as yet unstaled by use,
> The wonder of the ether had begun
> To fold the heavens up and reinduce
> That ancient hubris in the dreams of men,
> . . .
> —caution was absurd:
> Then let the ocean roll and the winds blow
> While the risk at Lloyds remained a record low.

The poet introduces the nemesis of the ship, "The Iceberg":

> Calved from a glacier near Godhaven coast,
> It left the fiord for the sea—a host
> Of white flotillas gathering in its wake,
> And joined by fragments from a Behring floe,
> Had circumnavigated to make
> It centre of an archipelago
> Its lateral motion on the Davis Strait
> Was casual and indeterminate,
> . . .
> No Smoke
> Of steamships nor the hoist of mainsails broke
> The polar wastes—no sounds except the grind
> Of ice,
> . . .
> It struck the current of the Labrador
> Which swung it to its definite southern stride.

*Pressure and glacial time had stratified*
*The berg to the consistency of flint,*
*. . . F*
*But with an impulse governed by the raw*
*Mechanics of its birth, it drifted where*
*Ambushed, fog—grey, it stumbled on its lair,*
*North forty-one degrees and forty-four,*
*Fifty and fourteen west the longitude,*
*Waiting a world-memorial hour, its rude*
*Corundum form stripped to its Greenland core.*

From the Bridge:

MURDOCH HOLDING THE BRIDGE—WATCH
*Starboard your helm:* ship heeled
*To port. From bridge to engine—room the clang*
*Of the telegraph. Danger. Stop. A hand sprang*
*To the throttle; the valves closed, and with the churn*
*Of the reverse the sea boiled at the stern.*
*Smith hurried to the bridge and Murdoch closed*
*The bulkheads of the ship as he supposed,*
*But could not know that with those riven floors*
*The electro-magnets failed upon the doors.*
*No shock! No more than if something alive*
*Had brushed her as she passed. The bow had missed.*
*Under the vast momentum of her drive*
*She went a mile. But why that ominous five*
*Degrees (within five minutes) of a list?*
*. . .*

From the Bridge

*As leaning on her side to ease a pain,*
*The tilted ship had stopped the captain's breath:*
*The inconceivable had stabbed his brain,*
*This thing unfelt—her visceral wound of death?*
*Another message—this time to report her*
*Filling, taxing the pumps beyond their strain.*
*Had that blow rent her from the bow to quarter?*
*Or would the aft compartments still intact*

*Give buoyancy enough to counteract*
*The open forward holds?*

The poem concludes:

*And out there in the starlight, with no trace*
*Upon it of its deed but the last wave*
*From the Titanic fretting at its base,*
*Silent, composed, ringed by its icy broods,*
*The grey shape with the paleolithic face*
*Was still the master of the longitudes.*[6]

Fascination with the sinking of the *Titanic* was emphasized by how much was unknown about the tragedy. What really caused it to sink and where on the seabed of the cold North Atlantic did it lie?

Down below in our cabin, I listened with trepidation to the sounds of ice scraping alongside the hull of the ship. This combined with the ship's constant back and forth motion gave rise to unpleasant thoughts and imagined scenarios, based on what I had viewed in the 1958 movie, *A Night to Remember*. Every one was a chilly reminder of those who had perished in the sinking of the *Titanic*. What would happen if the *Howe* was badly damaged by the ice? Would the bulkhead doors hold back the sea water from those sections damaged by the ice? Was rescue close at hand?

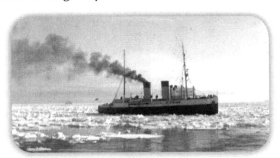

*This image of the* N.B. McLean, *under full power with black smoke streaming from her funnel, shows the extent of heavy pack ice. In the lower left corner, the churning wake from the screws of the* Howe *may be seen. Beyond the stern of the* McLean *is the* d'Iberville, *and off her bow, there is a freighter. Author's collection.*

---

6  Excerpts from "The Titanic," by E.J. Pratt, from *E.J. Pratt: Complete Poems*, edited by Sandra Djwa and R.G. Moyles, University of Toronto Press 1989. Reprinted with permission of the publisher.

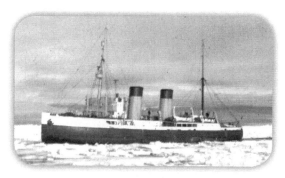

*CGS* N.B. McLean *clearing a passage through thick, heavy ice in Resolute Bay. A convoy, which included a freighter and a tanker, had to follow a passage made by the icebreakers. Author's collection.*

As the *Howe* drew closer to her destination, the helicopter was sent on ice reconnaissance in search of a safe passage through the ice. It was able to land at the Resolute Bay air base to pick up mail, but upon returning to the ship, the pilot reported that solid ice blanketed Resolute Bay. This meant further delays.

The *Howe* lay outside the bay awaiting favourable ice conditions.

Regardless, it was a welcome event to receive mail. I had been out of touch with family since leaving Churchill. The letters, packages, and newspapers from the home front brought good news, although none of recent events. Regardless, they eased my feelings of loneliness, and I returned to the cabin for some personal time to read and enjoy my mail.

My ship's papers were also included in this latest mail delivery. On the day I signed on, I was required to submit my official papers to the captain. I did not have them at that time, which created all sorts of ill-will with the captain, even more so after the ship received a radio signal from Ottawa confirming that I was approved as a cabin steward and assigned to the *Howe*.

I decided to take my papers to the purser, who was responsible for these matters. He had also expressed displeasure over my lack of papers, a situation he took pains to remind me of on those rare occasions we ran into each other. More discomfort.

"Come in," he announced after I knocked on his door. I entered the cabin and stood before him. I thought for sure he could see me tremble and read the fear written all over my face.

He was dressed in a casual uniform of white shirt and blue trousers. A short man, he had a hawkish face marked by a thin nose over thin lips. He threw me a hard, penetrating look, which I had difficulty avoiding. I felt he could scare the truth from you with little effort.

He sat behind his desk, which, to me, acted as a barrier between us and seemed to me a symbol of his rank.

Purser Brie spent several minutes looking me over. His sullen expression made it clear he wondered why I was here, taking up his valuable time.

"Mr. Brie, I apologize for interrupting." I tried to speak clearly, but the words seemed to get caught in my throat. "I have my papers authorizing my presence on board."

"Hand them over," Brie commanded. He flipped through my papers, scanning the contents, then propped his elbows on the desk.

"Okay, that is all for now. You may go." I was dismissed.

With that, I turned and left the purser's office, relieved that the encounter was finished. There had been no thanks, no recognition of producing my papers, as per regulations. Regardless, I had done my duty; now I was anxious to see what the effect would be, if any. I thought that by presenting my papers, the negative comments and harassment from the captain and the purser would end. Fat chance. Both men continued as they had begun.

The *Howe* dropped anchor in Resolute Bay, but large pans of ice extended out from the ship and covered the surface of the bay, making it impossible to launch the barges. It was August 14. The convoy comprising the CGS *N.B. McLean*, CGS *d'Iberville*, both icebreakers, and the two freighters was nowhere in sight. The CGS *Labrador*, an icebreaker usually deployed in the high Arctic waters, had encountered difficulties with the heavy ice conditions resulting in cracked plates. Her captain had decided to return to Quebec for repairs. Once again, navigating in northern waters had resulted in unexpected changes to itineraries.

The wind shifted overnight. While the bay was now clear of ice, there was still a lot of ice stacked up along the shoreline, which prevented the barges from landing. The helicopter transported

Eskimos from the *Howe* to the airport to be flown south to medical facilities.

The wind shifted in direction and velocity again, and large pans of ice drifted back into the bay. The barges were hoisted on board and secured. It was an amazing sight. I stood on the deck looking at the large ice floes as they floated into the bay. Within a short time, the ship was completely surrounded by and locked in ice.

The next day, activity on board had come to a halt. The ice surrounding the ship made it impossible to unload cargo. Chief Steward Moreau had plans to keep us busy.

The stewards department was ordered to clean the Eskimo quarters in the forward portion of the ship. These quarters were accessed through an upright hatch located just forward of the large crane. The area was smaller than a regular cargo hold, and there were portholes on the port and starboard sides. Alongside the bulkheads were several bunk beds, while in the centre was an open space for leisure activities.

The cleaning job, under the watchful eyes of the chief, took more than two hours to complete, even with the assistance of some of the seamen. They informed us that the Eskimo quarters were being converted to living/sleeping quarters for the soon-to-arrive contingent of stevedores. The seamen jokingly referred to the *Howe* as a "floating hotel." Upon completion, the quarters were in excellent shape in anticipation of the new arrivals.

The next day, Sunday, August 16, was beautiful. Out on deck, it was warm and the bright sun glistened off the ice. It was a sign that we do something special and take advantage of the fine, warm weather. While looking out over the ice, I was joined at the ship's rail by Robbie Levack, the helicopter pilot.

"How would you like a flip in the whirlybird?" he asked. "You and your cabin mates would get some time ashore." I thought this would be a welcome diversion and give us a chance to stretch our legs.

Robbie stated, "You need permission to leave the ship, first."

At just this moment, we were approached by Dr. Stevens, Officer-in-Charge, Eastern Arctic Patrol. Perfect. "Dr. Stevens, Robbie has offered to fly us ashore—a chance to explore and stretch our legs. May we have permission to go ashore?" I asked.

"Completely out of the picture. Captain's orders," Dr. Stevens replied tersely. So much for that little gambit. We could not see the reasoning behind this decision, other than something originating from the captain.

Although I continued chatting with Robbie and Dr. Stevens, I continued to think that the request was reasonable under the present conditions. Needless to say, I was disappointed. All the same, I recalled my oath of obedience from when I signed on.

Robbie said that occasionally when he was flying he would set the "bird" down on the top of a large hill and explore. He'd collected fossils from some of these explorations, which he had shown me on occasion.

"The next time I have some spare time I would like to walk to that hill just over the way, not too far from Resolute Bay," I said, pointing in the direction of the hill. "It does not seem to be very far away, I'm sure I could get there and back in short order."

"Not in your life!" retorted Robbie. "That hill is more than five miles away. How do you expect to walk over to the hill and get back to the ship in time for your shift?"

"You must be mistaken," I stated. "Surely, that hill is but a short distance away."

"Your eyes are deceiving you. Your mind tells you it is a short distance, because there are no trees."

"Okay. I'll take your word for it." I was somewhat disappointed, but happy to have my knowledge of the North expanded.

Later that day, four ships appeared on the horizon: CGS *N.B. McLean*, CGS *d'Iberville*, the freighter MV *Federal Voyager*, and the tanker MV *Irvingwood*. I had mixed feelings about the forthcoming changes to schedules and routines and accompanying additional duties that would result with the arrival of these ships.

The convoy was four days late. Neither the MV *Federal Voyager* nor the MV *Irvingwood* was fitted to handle the ice conditions; therefore, the *McLean* and *d'Iberville* assisted in breaking ice in the path of these ships. With the exception of the *d'Iberville*, all ships dropped anchor in the bay. The larger draught of the *d'Iberville* prevented it from accessing the shallower waters of the bay.

"We make the overtime!" Steward Leaping Louis bluntly stated.

What did this mean? From past experience, we knew we would be working extra hours, but the extent of the overtime was beyond our ken.

The chief steward had outlined our duties and work schedule at the beginning of the tour. We had been informed that there were expectations of additional work, but the extent of those additional hours had remained unknown.

The revised work schedule had us working in shifts over twenty-four hours each day.

We were informed that the newly arrived stevedores were from Montreal where they were confined in prison and were temporarily released from incarceration.

After several days of inactivity, while waiting for the ice to clear, the convoy's arrival marked a series of changes, resulting in an atmosphere of excitement and anticipation that swept through the ship. The stevedores were assigned to their shifts—twelve hours on, twelve hours off.

Added to our regular tasks of making up cabins and working in the pantry, we cabin boys were to serve the stevedores their midnight meal, around 1 a.m., and breakfast, at 4 a.m. This meant that we had to grab some shut-eye whenever we could. Thus, we were scheduled to work our regular eight-hour shift during the day plus shifts of serving meals throughout the night.

One night after dinner, Bill and I went to the tuck shop for goodies and then returned to our cabin, where we played several hands of cribbage before finishing off the day with a brief stroll around the deck. Bill mentioned that he was thinking of leaving the ship while at Resolute Bay. This surprised me. I assumed that if you signed on for the trip, you were required to stay until the patrol was completed. Bill was quite sure that it would be possible to leave from Resolute, as there were regular flights to the south.

I enjoyed Bill's company, and over the past six weeks, we had established a warm friendship. If Bill decided to take the opportunity to leave the ship here and fly home, I would be unhappy, to say the least. As there was no further discussion, I wrote a few letters and

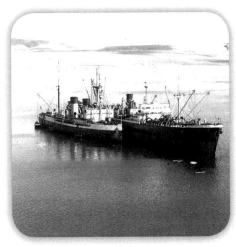

*CGS* N.B. McLean *alongside the freighter MV Federal Voyager.*
*Photo taken from helicopter. Photo courtesy of Dr. Ruth McLeese.*

went to bed, where I mulled over the possibility of Bill leaving and whether I should take this opportunity to return home, as well. Many thoughts, positive and negative, jumbled around my head as I dropped off into a restless sleep.

The next day, Monday, August 17, the weather was perfect. The barges were launched from the deck, seamen monitored the loading of cargo destined for Resolute Bay, and there was lots of activity about the ship; a determination to get the job done ASAP. Recent experience demonstrated that weather and ice conditions could change again, further delaying the scheduled tasks for this settlement.

The *N.B. McLean* ferried the stevedores from the freighter over to the *Howe*, where they would lodge for the duration of our stay in Resolute. I finished the wireless officer's cabin then went on deck to observe the activity. Securing the *McLean* alongside the *Howe* was a delicate operation, so as to avoid damaging the two ships, but was achieved without incident. Fortunately, the waters in the bay were calm, so the ships rode on their lines with only bumpers secured to the sides to keep them from rubbing against each other.

After the ships were secured, I joined up with my school chum, Mike Harris, from the *McLean*. We chatted about events since last meeting in Churchill, seemingly picking up where we had left off.

Shortly thereafter, seventy-four stevedores came on board. We assisted them with their luggage and got them settled in the former Eskimo quarters. At the same time, we had to assemble twenty sets of bunks and then make up forty beds. "Hotel *Howe*" had become a reality.

What a talkative group. As the chatter was all in French, I could not tell if they were expressing their displeasure with their new digs or their amazement with all the changes they were experiencing. I was certain their quarters were better than those they had left behind in Montreal. However, the atmosphere soon took on the semblance of "first day at summer camp," as they jostled to claim bunks and get settled in.

The *McLean,* having discharged the stevedores, slipped her ties to the *Howe,* and with sadness, I waved goodbye to Mike as his ship moved slowly away out into the bay. We both knew we probably would not see each other until we were back at home.

After a quick lunch in the mess, news came that the helicopter from the *d'Iberville* was transporting a crew member requiring medical attention. To my complete surprise, who should disembark but Bill Watters, another school chum. He had an abscessed tooth and was experiencing considerable pain. I went with him to the medical quarters.

A year behind me, Bill Watters and I lived in the same neighbourhood, chummed around in the same group of friends, and attended the same school, where we both enjoyed sports. He was a fast runner and enjoyed some notoriety in track and field competitions. A touch of home from "out of the blue."

At the dental office, Dr. Smithurst removed the offending tooth, while I waited in the outer area. Dr. Smithurst informed Bill that he would experience a few days of lingering pain, but he would soon be as good as new.

We then went to the Executive Suite, where we caught up on the news from home. He and I shared our feelings of homesickness and isolation, an effect of the North's vast expanse.

Bill W. was a seaman on the *d'Iberville,* so he took an interest in accompanying me as I completed my cabins. After he returned to his ship, I returned to the Suite to write some letters. I wanted to let family and friends know of the big events of this day. Bill's visit had been a breath of fresh air, bearing more news from home.

After dinner, I went up on deck again to enjoy some more of

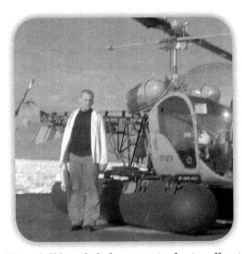

*Bill Kendall beside helicopter. Author's collection.*

the magnificent weather. The first mate, Mr. Pelletier, was there, too. I approached him and requested permission to go ashore on one of the barges. To my surprise, he agreed, then stated that the next barge going ashore was at 7 p.m., with the last return at 11 p.m. I conveyed this good news to my cabin mates, Bill and Sandy, and we went up on deck to board one of the barges. This was our first time off the ship since Churchill. Not necessarily a night on the town, but a time to visit friends we knew who had summer jobs on the military base located in Resolute.

Resolute Bay was a busy settlement of Eskimos and southerners. Some Eskimos lived in housing on the base while those who still lived a nomadic lifestyle were in tents for the summer. Southerners comprised people stationed at the Department of Transport weather station, a United States Weather Base, and the Royal Canadian Air Force base. The airport was located not far from the base housing facilities.

We were met at the shoreline by more school friends, Peter Brown, John McDiarmid, Jim Harvey, and John Watt, who took us up to the base for a tour. I was impressed by the large cafeteria, which was needed to feed the significant number of people stationed here, as part of the Cold War.

Afterwards, we went to Pete's cabin. Sitting around in this small room, we had an extended gabfest, as we caught up with everyone's comings and goings, news from home, and jobs. The chaps on base received mail regularly by air, so were way ahead of those of us at sea, who received news from home on an intermittent basis.

We then toured the base some more. We passed by the Eskimo housing and their tents, then beyond to the Resolute Bay Garbage Dump. We had been advised not to get too close to this "historic site" for security reasons. Every bit of waste generated at the settlement was deposited here, and while we did not get close enough to encounter any foul smells, we did see a plane fuselage. It was from a DC-3, an old cargo plane that had crashed on landing many years ago. As there was little left to salvage, it had been tossed into the garbage dump.

All too soon, our evening came to an end, and we made our way back to the rendezvous point for the return trip by barge. The fading rays from the sun setting in the west combined with the reflection of the full moon on the surface of the bay made a short, routine trip from shore to ship unforgettable.

Over the next several days, we maintained a steady schedule of making up cabins, cleaning the common area latrines, and, of course, executing pantry duty, the latter a mind-numbing task. Added to these tasks was waiting on tables twice each night for the stevedores. I was "making the overtime."

"Hold on a minute," shouted the first mate, Mr. Pelletier. I was on deck for a short break observing the activities. "Would you be willing to work overtime on cargo?"

"What does it involve?" I asked. I already had extra work and was leery about taking on more.

"I need some extra help alongside the seamen unloading cargo from the ship destined for this site," he said.

"Okay," I said. This would be an opportunity to go ashore and blow out some of the cobwebs that had accumulated working while in cramped spaces. I would also get a closeup view of the beach and landing areas.

"If you have finished your current tasks, get some warm clothes on, your boots, too, and meet at the barge to go ashore. The seamen will have some work gloves for you."

The seamen on the barge greeted me with smiles all round, which made me feel welcome, although I still was not sure what I had gotten myself into.

As we beached, I jumped off the barge on to the gravelly shore, where I almost fell over as I stumbled to get my footing. The many-coloured stones on the beach had been worn smooth and slippery by the water, making it difficult to stand. I gave a thought to explorers and whalers of past centuries who had also walked on this shore (curiosity never wanes), and noted the clarity of the water. It looked inviting enough to drink, even though I knew it was salt. I wondered if, given warmer weather, one might venture to take a swim. I put my hand in up to my elbow. At first it felt refreshing, but shortly after my arm went numb. I remembered then that the ice had only just receded from the bay. It was chilly!

"Listen up, men," the first mate commanded our attention. "Get the gangplank set up and start unloading. Be sure to put the cargo on the beach beyond the high tide mark." Here we go! I got in line to haul cargo, starting with huge bags of coal and flour.

Jeepers, they were heavy. I was nearly knocked off my feet when one of the seamen threw a bag of coal over my shoulder, and I am sure he was testing me, a cabin boy, to see if I could make the grade, carrying it down the gangplank to the designated place on shore. After a few faltering steps, I learned how to adjust the load. It did not take long to become accustomed to the rigours of this job.

Visibly surprised that I had not crumbled under the weight of the load, nor lost my footing, the seamen grinned widely as they bantered back and forth, *en français*, hoping this cabin boy would trip, fall on his face, and spill the load. That was NOT going to happen. Soon the seamen had established a rhythm, including me as one of them.

After a few days of the new schedule, we were exhausted. Between our regular duties during the day and extra duties serving the stevedores in the mess at night, there was little opportunity for sleep, let alone free time.

After our regular evening meal, Bill and I went up on to the Promenade Deck to get a breath of fresh air and take in the scenery. To our complete surprise, we were requested to assist carrying the baggage belonging to the four francophone cabin boys and a seaman who were leaving the ship. My recent discussion with Bill doing this very same thing flashed through my mind. This was sudden. There had been no scuttlebutt concerning this departure from the patrol. Surely there was a back story, but we didn't know it.

The ship's complement of cabin boys had, without warning, been cut in half. We realized that this reduction in staff would mean almost continual duty shifts throughout every twenty-four-hour period. Given time for meals and four-hour stints for sleep, there would be no time for shore leave and visits with our friends. It didn't matter; I was so tired I could not even think of going ashore.

The cargo work continued, but the cabin boys were not asked to pitch in and help. Then the wind shifted and the ice floes returned, bringing cargo unloading to a complete halt. The Bridge reported that ice coverage was 10/10,[7] meaning that as far as one could see from the deck, the bay was covered by a solid blanket of ice. This was a blessing in disguise, at least for us, as the stevedores could not work; therefore, we did not have to work nights. We reverted to our normal duties and tried to catch up on our sleep.

We had been at sea for eight weeks. This respite from our busy schedule would last as long as the ice kept the ship locked in. It was interesting to note that in about a month's time we would be back home. Some rumours amongst the men in the mess indicated we might be in Quebec City around September 25. To a certain extent, this was encouraging, as it gave us an end date to the journey. However, someone pointed out not to get one's hopes up. Surprises were more the norm than the exception in the North.

When I bumped into the first mate on deck as he was taking in the sights, I asked if he could confirm this arrival date.

"As you may know, this was the date posted on the itinerary circulated to all concerned in early June," replied Mr. Pelletier in a friendly, but guarded tone. "However, the emergency at Resolution Island has caused us to alter our plans. But given sailing conditions, I still predict our arrival on September 25. I know the captain and other officers are working towards this goal."

---

7  Ice concentration ratio describes how much a 10 x 10 mile area is covered by sea ice, ranging from 1/10 for open water, to 10/10 for compact, or consolidated ice.

As I returned to the cabin, I wondered what I should write and tell my parents about our date of arrival in Quebec. Ah! The vagaries of travelling in the North.

During my shifts in the pantry, I noticed that The Bass was upset. I did not want to inquire as to the cause, as it was probably none of my business. However, although he continued to address me as "my friend," I knew enough to say little, agree when questioned, or otherwise keep out of his way.

Nerves were frayed; verbal exchanges were curt; the ship continued to be icebound. There was lots of grumbling under one's breath, as one continued, somewhat grudgingly, to carry out assignments.

Finally, on the morning of the fifth day, there was a significant change in the direction and velocity of the wind. Looking out from the ship over the bay, all I could see was open water. The ice had gone, meaning it was back to work and a return to previous schedules for all. Cargo operations at the *Howe*, as well as the freighter and the oil tanker, resumed in earnest and with enthusiasm.

The ship's officers, anxious to get caught up, pushed the timetable. One of the seamen, Jean-Marc Thibideau, badly injured his leg during cargo operations, which sent him to the ship's hospital. I went to visit him that evening. I had befriended Jean-Marc during cargo work. He was a large, strong, jovial fellow and

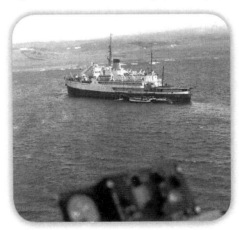

*Howe from chopper, with barges and hydrographic launches alongside.*
*Photo courtesy of Dr. Ruth McLeese.*

had readily accepted me on the cargo team. He was feeling better, but still in a lot of pain. I wished him a speedy recovery.

The next day, operations continued, as did the routine chores. As ever, I was doing my best in the pantry, washing dishes and cutlery while avoiding the two stewards and their snide comments (in French), which I had no difficulty understanding.

Meanwhile, I wondered what would happen to the empty oil barrels and other used materials. I asked the stevedores while serving their midnight meal, and they replied that they would load the empty oil barrels and other miscellaneous items into the cargo holds of the freighter, where they would be transported to a southern port for further disposal. Mystery solved.

The stevedores often joked with us while we served their meals and expressed their appreciation for the good food through their hearty appetites.

After a couple hours of sleep, I was awakened to go to the mess hall and again serve the stevedores. After a quick breakfast at 7 a.m., the chief steward ordered us to the Eskimo quarters. The stevedores had packed their belongings and had proceeded to the barges for transportation ashore. They would fly back to Montreal.

In addition to cleaning the entire area that had housed the stevedores, we had to store the extra bunks, rearrange the remaining bunks, and make up the beds. The living quarters were in tip-top shape again for the new intake of Eskimos.

On completion of these tasks, I went to make up those cabins assigned to me. I was very tired, so I was slow in getting them done. At noon, I was on duty in the pantry, where I suspected that stewards Leaping Louis and The Bass were also tired. I could also tell that The Bass was quite upset; you could cut the atmosphere in there with a knife. A man of few kind words at the best of times, I was careful not to incur further anger, either from him or Leaping Louis, as they snipped at each other. I could not wait until this shift was over.

After the hectic pace of our two weeks in Resolute Bay, I was ready for a break. Fortunately, I was able to get ashore and visit with friends, but the respite was short-lived.

In a month's time, we were scheduled to dock in Quebec City. In the meantime, I looked forward to our arrival at Arctic Bay and then, our most northerly destination, Grise Fiord.

# Chapter Ten

# Grise Fiord, Ellesmere Island, Jones Sound

As the *Howe* departed Resolute Bay and sailed eastward in Lancaster Sound, progress was slow and various courses were followed to seek safe passage through the heavy ice. Although we continued with our regular tasks, the long hours and limited sleep over the past two weeks had taken their toll. Soon after the evening meal, we retired to our cabin. Sleep came quickly.

The next day brought a welcome change in both the weather and our spirits. The sun shone brightly, and the waters of Admiralty Inlet were clear of ice. It promised to be a terrific day.

As the *Howe* slowly approached the tiny settlement of Arctic Bay, I grabbed my camera and stepped out onto the port side of the

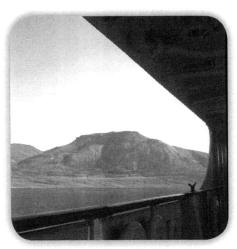

*King Mountain, Arctic Bay. Author's collection*

Promenade Deck to get the best possible view. Off in the distance, I could see a high hill known as King Mountain, which towered over the tiny settlement. Halfway up the hill, the settlement's name, Arctic Bay, was spelled out in stones painted white, while along the shore was a cluster of buildings, also white. The contrast of brown earth and blue sea made for a picture-perfect scene.

All aboard were busy performing their duties. The sunny weather had an uplifting effect on our efforts.

It had been a few days since I had last visited with Jean-Marc in sick bay. We chatted about the fine weather, the fact that most on board were pleased to have completed the sojourn at Resolute Bay, and what to expect during the next section of the tour. It was great that Jean-Marc was feeling much better.

The next morning, I was back in the pantry. Many had yet to come to the dining salon, but my orders were to remain. It was shaping up to be a lengthy shift, not made any easier by The Bass's continued bad humour, which he took out on me. Word soon got out that there had been a real shindig last night that had lasted until the wee small hours.

The captain passed the pantry door, and I could see a seaman assisting him navigate the narrow passageway to the dining salon for a late breakfast. He appeared unstable on his feet, and I noticed he was sporting a large purple goose egg in the middle of his forehead. Apparently, he had bumped his head on a steel bulkhead, or at least that was the official explanation.

Shortly thereafter, more passengers appeared in the salon for breakfast, or, more accurately, brunch.

Alas, our stay in Arctic Bay was altogether too short. Given the fine weather and the picturesque setting, I thought it would be grand to spend more time there. We weighed anchor for our next port of call, Grise Fiord, located on the southerly tip of Ellesmere Island.

At a much reduced speed, we left Lancaster Sound and entered into Baffin Bay. Our course northward was plagued by heavy ice floes, which covered a large portion of the water surface.

Those passing close to the ship were estimated to be eight to twelve feet thick, with mounds of snow on the top. They were blue, almost turquoise in colour, and were different from those seen earlier, during our southerly travels in Hudson Strait and Lancaster Sound. Also in this ice field were lots of "bergy bits," so-called by the seamen, but no icebergs.

These "bergy bits" referred to large pieces of irregularly shaped ice chunks that had broken off icebergs. They had a higher profile than the flat-topped ice floes we had observed in our earlier travels. The "bergy bits," seen up close, had a significant, deep underwater profile. They came from glaciers and, therefore, were a source of fresh water; a couple of chunks in your cocktail was a special treat.

The scenery of Devon Island was breathtaking, and I was overwhelmed by this majestic panorama. Beyond the shoreline was the flat, brownish terrain that rose up to form rocky, brownish-grey hills. Higher up, these hills were covered with snow and ice; white clouds provided the icing on top. This view was engraved in my mind. A treasure of the high north.

The *Howe* navigated a passage through the heavy polar ice. Helicopter reconnaissance reported the ice pack extended in a thirty-mile radius around the *Howe*. Fortunately, the ship could follow along the edge of the ice pack, and we continued sailing in a northerly direction. We left the ice pack behind as the ship sailed into Jones Sound.

I ran into Mr. Laxton, the wireless/radio officer, as he was leaving his cabin and going to the Bridge. After exchanging pleasantries, I asked him about the ships on the horizon I had seen over the past few days. They looked like black specks floating on the horizon and appeared to be shadowing us.

"Those are Russian trawlers," replied Mr. Laxton. "They have been keeping an eye on us for a number of days, as well as listening to our radio communications. Ottawa has been informed and has ordered us to maintain radio silence."

While I knew about the Cold War, this was the first time I had ever really encountered it. How closely were we being watched? Were there any Soviet spies on those trawlers? Could there be an international incident in this isolated part of Canada? This was a chilling introduction to the reality of world politics.

Grise Fiord, situated on the southern tip of Ellesmere Island, had held a special fascination for me throughout the trip. Our furthest destination north, and now I was here. My first reaction was to be awestruck by the majestic grandeur of the setting. There was a buildup of ice along the shore, probably drifted in, with three or four buildings scattered along the shoreline. Mountains towered over this small community. The overall effect was one of serenity.

We arrived in Grise Fiord on Sunday, August 30. As we sailed into the bay approaching the anchorage, a few Eskimos along the shore waved, with broad grins on their faces. The RCMP contingent was also out in full force—all two officers. The annual visit by the *Howe* was a special time for all. There was an expectation of supplies for the coming year and contact with others "from away." The ship took on a sense of urgency, so as to make the most of the declining hours of warmth and sunlight to unload the cargo and distribute special packages, food parcels, and mail.

Once again, the first mate asked if I wanted to work on cargo. I readily agreed, as it meant I would get to go ashore; I quickly went to join the first loaded barge. The beach was similar to the one at Resolute Bay, composed of many small, round stones and pebbles. Getting a foothold was tricky; the smooth stones would roll under one's feet. I quickly scanned the beach, hoping that I might find something to serve as a souvenir. No luck. We were ordered to bend our shoulders to the job, as it had to be completed before the tide ebbed. The Eskimos joined in to give us a hand, while the RCMP officers took on the clerical responsibilities of recording the goods and their disposition. The Eskimos yapped amongst themselves, with a few "yaps" directed our way. We may not have understood what they were saying, but we appreciated their "EEEs" of happiness, which made the work progress quickly. All too soon the job was completed, and we boarded the barge and returned to the ship.

Following lunch, I resumed my regular duties in the pantry then completed my cabins. The weather this day was excellent, with the settlement bathed in bright, warm sunshine, disturbed by only a few clouds and a light breeze. I spent some time up on the Bridge Deck on my way to W/T Officer Laxton's cabin. The view from there was so spectacular that it took my breath away. I could see the high hills stretching along the horizon, the shoreline where we unloaded cargo, and the few small buildings nestled at the base of the hills.

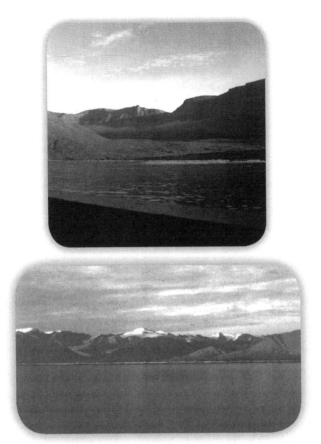

*Grise Fiord at sunset. Author's collection.*

In 1993, I caught an interview with Dr. Shelagh D. Grant by Peter Gzowski on CBC Radio's *Morningside*, discussing the relocation of Eskimo families from Port Harrison to Grise Fiord (Craig Harbour) in 1953; CGS *C.D. Howe* was the ship used to effect the move.

The interview discussed several aspects of the relocation and revealed hardships faced by the inhabitants, who were left to fend for themselves in the new location. When I arrived at Grise Fiord, these were the Eskimos who welcomed the *Howe* so warmly. They had been living there for six years. The following is an example of the families who came and what they brought with them:[8]

---

8   Shelagh D. Grant, "A Case of Compounded Error: The Inuit Resettlement Project, 1953, and the Government Response, 1990," *Northern Perspectives* (Canadian Arctic Resources Committee) Vol 19, Number 1 (Spring 1991), p.17.

- 1 hunter, wife, 1 son, 2 daughters, 1 sled, 5 dogs, 2 rifles, 20 traps, 1 tent, 1 kayak

- 1 hunter, 3 sons, 1 daughter, 1 sled, 5 dogs, 1 rifle, 20 traps, a tent, a kayak

Grise Fiord was the northernmost settlement in Canada. The sun sets in October and does not appear above the horizon until April—a long winter of darkness. With the limited communications of the day, there must have been a deep sense of isolation there. The terrain has little vegetation for use as either food or fuel. Recalling my memories of the settlement, I realized that the relocation must have been fraught with difficulties and hardships.

The Eskimos revealed themselves to be a hardy lot. They worked together and, with their diligence and survival skills, created a community. Their smiles, chatter, and infectious laughter as they boarded the *Howe* for their medical examinations proved to me that they made the best of things. They extended this community spirit to us by assisting in the unloading of cargo. While this assistance may have been self-serving, as they anticipated

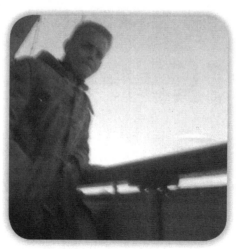

*At Grise Fiord, an Eskimo boy approached us and asked if he could look at my camera. At first, I was reluctant to agree, fearing he might damage it or throw it overboard, but I soon gave in, and he immediately took this picture of Bill Kendall. We all had a good laugh, before he left to rejoin his family. Author's collection.*

receiving some of the contents of the cargo for themselves, I took it to mean that all was well with them and their community.

All operations were completed by mid-afternoon, and the anchor was raised. Knowing that the *Howe* would not return until next year, the departure was bittersweet. I thought we would be here longer. Such was not the case, as there were many communities yet to visit on the *Howe*'s schedule. Grise Fiord, with the Eskimos and RCMP officers waving goodbye, slowly diminished as we sailed out the bay. To this day, I can visualize the fading sight of this small community in Canada's far north.

# Chapter Eleven

# Pond Inlet,
# Baffin Island

**W**ith memories of my final glimpses of the Grise Fiord settlement tucked away, I turned my mind to Pond Inlet, the next community on the itinerary. During the night, as we sailed past three Eskimo camps, the helicopter ferried Eskimos to and from the ship for their medical checkups. Dr. Oschinsky requested my assistance recording anthropological information. We completed the survey about 2 a.m., and I returned to the cabin for a few hours of welcome sleep.

That afternoon, after completing routine duties, I joined my fellow cabin mates to polish brass. Was another special event scheduled with invited guests? Afterwards, I ventured out on the

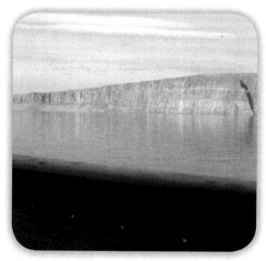

*Bylot Island, off Baffin Island. Author's collection.*

Promenade Deck. I had heard rumours that Pond Inlet was the most scenic in the North, so I wanted to see for myself whether there was any truth in these tales.

As we sailed through a narrow waterway towards Pond Inlet, on the starboard side I saw the massive rock face of Bylot Island.

I was awestruck. It was truly beautiful. The settlement was surrounded by mountains, glaciers, and ice floes. Sun dappled on the waters of the inlet, where fishing boats bobbed at anchor. Along the shore, I could see the Hudson's Bay Company store, the RCMP building, and the Catholic church, all wood-framed buildings painted white with red metal roofs, which gave the community a unified look. The rumours were right; Pond Inlet was a jewel of the North.

Then, suddenly, it seemed as though the entire community was scurrying to the shoreline to greet our arrival. Eskimo men, women (some with babies in their hoods), children, RCMP officers, Hudson's Bay post administrators, and members of the clergy waved joyously as the *Howe* approached its anchorage. The dogs joined in the welcome, barking and dashing about the feet of those gathered. An unbelievable atmosphere of happiness prevailed. I considered myself most fortunate to see the exuberance of the people gathered at the shoreline.

All too soon, I had to return to the pantry to prepare for a dinner planned for that evening. Undoubtedly, the *Howe* would be hosting guests from Pond Inlet.

My shipboard duties completed, I was asked to assist the seamen with cargo. It was eight o'clock in the evening, and the temperature outside was dropping, so I dressed quickly in warm clothes and boots to go ashore. I could hear the chugging noise of the engine on the barge; it was fully loaded, and there was just room enough for me and a few others. We finished our shift at one o'clock in the morning, working under lights from the ship once the sun set. The work was strenuous, but it kept us warm. Back on ship, I went down to the cabin, anxious to get some shut-eye, as I knew I would be back on cargo duty in a few hours. The changes in the tide dictated our working hours.

After four hours of sleep, I again donned warm clothes and boarded the landing barge. Under the keen eye of the first mate, we were pressed to get the job done in short order. We needed little urging; although the sun had risen, the temperature on the beachhead was only 43°F.

One incident that brought laughter to the ship's crew and the Eskimos assisting us occurred while unloading a cumbersome wooden building frame from the barge.

A narrow plank had been placed between the barge and the shoreline, which we used to carry the supplies from the barge onto shore. I noticed that while the water was shallow near the shore, after a few feet, it dropped off abruptly.

After several trips, during which we had unloaded numerous hundred-pound sacks of food and forty-five-gallon oil drums, it was time to transport a number of large wooden building frames. The barge came as close to shore as its draught would allow and then the narrow gangplank was set up. There was just enough room on the plank for one person to traverse in single file. However, the heavy, awkward frames required two people, one on each side, to manoeuvre them down the plank to the shore. Despite the challenge, we managed, with the assistance of some of the Eskimos. Among those helping was a tall, husky, Eskimo man, with a big, booming voice. While ably hoisting two sacks at a time onto his shoulders, he cracked jokes, to all of the Eskimos' amusement, and those on shore began laughing and pointing fingers. He was obviously enjoying the attention his strength and wit were garnering.

With the urging of his friends, the big Eskimo grabbed one side of a building frame, while his partner grabbed the other. It was obvious by the determined look on his face that he was intent on proving that he could do just about anything. Together, they shuffled down the plank, the big Eskimo walking backwards, carefully placing one foot behind the other. Everyone was laughing and yelling at him to watch his step. He paid little notice to the taunts, as he was more concerned with keeping his balance. As luck would have it, just before reaching shore, his foot slipped off the plank and he dropped the frame. He was now knee-deep, with the water pouring over the top of his rubber boots. On taking stock of his predicament, however, he burst out laughing and started sloshing to shore. Soon, everyone was laughing—the Eskimos, the ship's crews, and even those who had come to see what had happened.

The Eskimos enjoyed a good laugh, particularly if it involved one of their friends in a mishap or pratfall. Sometimes, the laughter reached a point where any and all tasks at hand were forgotten, as the incident was recounted and replayed, again and again. This was such an occasion. The big Eskimo did not seem put out by what had happened. In fact, his friends came up and patted him on the back, clearly demonstrating that they were laughing with him, not at him.

What a memory. Even to this day, I can still see clearly in my mind's eye our big friend slipping off the plank and falling into the cold sea water, and hear the laughter as it spread amongst the crowd, Eskimo and southerner alike.

This day marked the first time in many weeks that I did not have pantry duty. My first reaction was that I would not have to work alongside The Bass, who continued to make snide remarks. What a relief. While I did not keep track as to how many hours I had served in the pantry, I knew I had spent significantly more time there than my cabin mates. So be it. I hoped I would not have to return to the odious job of scullery maid in the company of those who did nothing but verbally abuse me.

Shortly after lunch, there was a stir of activity. "Admiral" Tubbe, a seaman, had become stranded on one of the barges, which had slipped its moorings. The Admiral was responsible for fitting out the barge so that it could be winched aboard and secured on the deck. He was a large, self-important man, who made sure everyone knew it, hence the nickname "Admiral." He may have even perceived himself as captain of the barge. Anyway, the situation was quickly remedied, and Admiral Tubbe was saved from further embarrassment.

Our visit to Pond Inlet was coming to an end. Unfortunately, I had had no time during this short stopover to take any pictures of this very picturesque settlement.

My last view of Pond Inlet was the crowd of Eskimos on the beachhead waving their goodbyes. Although I was very tired, I was also a bit sad; this image will remain with me for all time.

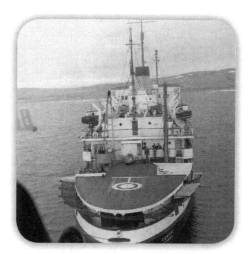

*Helicopter landing on stern pad. Note the two hydrographic launches in the stern davits on the Boat Deck. Photo courtesy of Dr. Ruth McLeese.*

We had been at sea for ten weeks, yet still had many communities to visit. In the next twenty-four-hour period, we would visit Scott Inlet and Sam Ford Fiord where, again, the Eskimos were transported by helicopter to and from the ship for the medical survey. I carried on with my regular duties, and although I was on standby for cargo work, I was not called; a heavy easterly swell made it impossible to unload cargo.

We arrived at Clyde River early Friday morning, September 4. It was a cool, overcast day with some periods of rain. First Mate Pelletier asked that I join the crew to work cargo; we commenced work shortly after 1 p.m. We carried heavy sacks of flour and sugar, and rolled forty-five-gallon drums of oil up to the site. It was hard work. Often, we would work in pairs. Most of the seamen spoke only French, but I muddled through, enjoying at least the camaraderie of the seamen. Our short conversations helped make the work go faster and seem easier, until the tide had ebbed to a point where the barges were too far from shore.

At 10 p.m., I had a light lunch then returned to my station on shore to continue unloading cargo. The tide had turned, making it possible to access the shore, but the sun had long set. It was pitch black out, with the exception of a few lights shining on board the ship and on shore, powered by the settlement's generator. We continued working until 5 a.m., when the tide again ebbed; in fuel alone, we had unloaded and rolled ashore 800 drums.

"I have made good friends with all the seamen . . . it's a real ball . . . it's cool working on the beachhead but we are kept warm by working . . ." I wrote in my diary.

I woke up shortly after eight-thirty that same morning, groggy from lack of sleep and with little energy to tackle routine tasks. However, I was assured that the community was grateful of our efforts. These supplies were to last them until next year.

Today, a wedding was celebrated on board, with the officer-in-charge conducting the ceremony. Later in the afternoon, the reception was held in the dining salon. I knew nothing of these events until after the fact.

It occurred to me that this was extraordinary, but then life in the North was nothing but extraordinary.

# Chapter Twelve

# Cape Christian to Cape Dyer, Baffin Island, Davis Strait

The *Howe* proceeded southward along the east coast of Baffin Island. The weather was favourable for smooth sailing at cruising speed, and Davis Strait was free of ice; therefore, no sooner did we arrive at one settlement then we were on to the next. Some settlements had few inhabitants; one, in fact, had only two families.

On the Promenade Deck, I leaned over the ship's rail and followed the patterns of the bow waves. The bow was slicing through the water as she steamed onward, creating white, frothing waves that spread out from the bow, while the wake bubbled up behind us, marking our passage through the clear waters.

I continued with my regular duties, taking frequent breaks on the Promenade Deck to catch glimpses of the eastern coast of Baffin Island. Now that we were heading south, the *Howe* seemed to be travelling quickly. My feelings were mixed, as I realized that the patrol was nearing its end and we would soon be home.

There was a rumour circulating on board that we could be ordered back to Churchill. While it was doubtful that this would be the case, that did not stop the speed of the "news" as it travelled around the ship. I dared not ask the wireless operator, Mr. Laxton, as this was Bridge business—not mine. There were quite a few settlements left to visit on our itinerary, and the thought of returning to Churchill was demoralizing. I trusted that we would continue on our present course.

Below is a chart of the settlements the *Howe* visited, no matter how short the visit, and some were very short. However, regardless of the time of arrival, the medical survey was conducted. Note also that we crossed the Arctic Circle on more than one occasion (66° 5′ N), albeit there was no fanfare on subsequent crossings. As the *Howe* sailed southward, the sun set earlier in the evening and rose later in the morning. These changes, as well as the weather, signalled we were leaving the North.

| Eskimo Settlement | Date | Latitude | Arrival | Departure |
|---|---|---|---|---|
| Cape Christian | Sept 6 | 69° 38′ N | 03:30:00 | 04:30:00 |
| Ekalugad Fiord | Sept 7 | 68° 29′ N | 01:30:00 | 15:00:00 |
| Cape Hooper | Sept 7 | 68° 29′ N | 09:30:00 | 11:30:00 |
| Kivitoo | Sept 7 | 68° 29′ N | 19:30:00 | 08:30:00 |
| Broughton Island | Sept 8 | 67° 35′ N | 01:30:00 | 18:30:00 |
| Padloping Island | Sept 9 | 66° 48′ N | 01:30:00 | 06:30:00 |
| Durban Island | Sept 9 | 66° 48′ N | 08:15:00 | 09:00:00 |
| Cape Dyer | Sept 9 | 66° 48′ N | 15:00:00 | 18:15:00 |

By now, I was familiar with most areas of the ship. I had explored the forward holds, galleys and messes, the bridge, the radio room, and the engine room. However, I had not been to the cargo area in the stern on the Main Deck, located three decks below the helicopter landing pad. This section of the ship had been off limits. However, as this area was now empty, I decided to take a surreptitious tour, so that I could watch the moonbeams dance on the calm surface of the sea.

As I stepped onto the deck, I marvelled at the sight of the shimmering white wake as it disappeared into the blackness of the night. However, beyond the wake, there was nothing. NOTHING. There was no evidence we had cut a path through the water. Who would know that we had been here?

I slowly moved towards the stern of the ship. I wanted to see the full expanse of the night sky, which was blocked by the deck above. On this clear night, I could easily find the North Star, the Milky Way, and the Big and Little Dippers, plus a myriad other stars I had no idea even existed. Their beauty was diminished only by the light of the moon.

I looked towards the coast of Baffin Island, draped in ghostly shadows.

I heard the rumble of the engines below and felt the vibration of the propellers as they churned through the water. I noticed the deck was wet, probably from mist in the air and the spray from the bow waves. I needed to take caution, as a single misstep could easily result in my slipping into the sea, with no one the wiser.

Here I was.

> *The Arctic trails have their secret tales*
> *That would make your blood run cold;*

—Robert W. Service, "The Cremation of Sam McGee"

# Chapter Thirteen

# Pangnirtung, Baffin Island, Cumberland Sound

I was awakened early on September 10 by the loud, scraping sound of ice as the *Howe* slowly made her way through a wide expanse of ice floes. I got out of bed and placed my hand on the interior skin of the ship. I could feel as well as hear the ice scraping against the steel hull; it was eerie. A thin sheet of steel was all that separated me from the powerful ice floes. The noise reverberated through our small cabin as the ship negotiated its way through yet another ice field.

After breakfast, I went out to the starboard rail on the Promenade Deck and where I discovered that we were surrounded

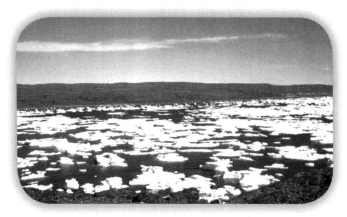

*"Bergy bits" in Frobisher Bay. From the Delaute family collection, courtesy of E. (Liz) Delaute Simms.*

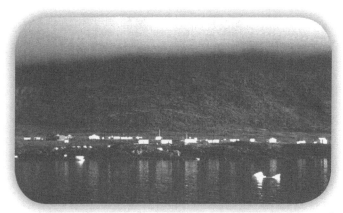

*Pangnirtung, Cumberland Sound, under a dense cloud. Author's collection.*

by heavy, but loose ice. Scattered amongst the ice were several "bergy bits."

Before long, however, we sailed out of the ice field, and in the distance, I could make out the greyish, rocky coastline. It was a stunning sight—deep blue water and wall-to-wall sun. If I did not know I was in the North, I would think I was sailing on one of the Great Lakes.

In the far distance, I could see something silver hugging the coast. Upon inquiry, I learned that this was a DEW Line station, part of a system of radar stations throughout the North and another reminder of the ongoing Cold War.

We dropped anchor at Pangnirtung at 6:30 p.m., just after our evening meal. Above the beachhead standing on the escarpment, a group of Eskimos welcomed us with shouts of warm greetings and the waving of arms. It was a sight I had seen previously at other settlements. Just the same, it was a pleasure to see and experience this good cheer again. It looked as though some were so happy to see us that they were dancing about. Their dogs were getting into the welcoming routine, too, by running about. In retrospect, I am sure the warm welcome was more likely in honour of the anticipated arrival of much-needed goods, supplies, fuel, and mail. The yearly visit of the *Howe* was an important and festive event, and a holiday atmosphere was apparent before we reached shore.

Shortly after the anchor was lowered and set, the barges were launched for the transferring of cargo to the settlement. Pangnirtung had more than 500 Eskimos, making it one of the larger communities in the Eastern Arctic. The medical team would be busy, as would I, helping with cargo.

The next day, cargo work began early. After a quick breakfast, we climbed aboard a barge filled with supplies. We discovered that the beach consisted of the same multicoloured stones we had experienced at previous landings. Once again, I stepped cautiously while shouldering heavy sacks of flour and sugar. These supplies had to be transported to the top of the cliff. This was a difficult job, but with help from some of the Eskimos, it progressed well. The work was also made lighter by the Eskimos' continuous chatter and laughter. By noon, the tide began to ebb, and we climbed on board the barge to return to the ship. After lunch, I went to our cabin for a short but needed rest.

I then returned to my regular shipboard duties of cleaning the passenger cabins and public latrines. In the late afternoon, I went up on deck, where I had a pleasant chat with the first mate, Mr. Pelletier.

"With this stop and a few more, we should be able to make our ETA in Quebec City on the 25th of September, just as you had predicted in one of our earlier chats."

"Yes, I believe I can confirm that prediction," he replied. "But remember, there is still a lot of cargo work to do, and you never can tell what will happen between now and then."

I was pleased and encouraged by this information. I could now write to my parents informing them of this welcome news.

While we were still more than ten days from Quebec, I had no reason to doubt the first mate. He had many years of experience on the Eastern Arctic Patrol and had always been straight with me.

I was looking forward to the end of the patrol. I had not received mail since Resolute Bay three weeks ago, and my thoughts had begun to focus on home.

After the evening meal, I was informed the tide had turned; therefore, if I wanted to work on cargo, the barge was going ashore in fifteen minutes. I dashed down to the cabin and dressed in my warm work clothes and boots. Up on deck, I prepared to climb aboard the barge with other seamen and Sandy Bryce, a cabin mate.

It was going on eight o'clock in the evening, and the sun had set. Once we unloaded the cargo from the barge, it returned to the ship for another load. The process of reloading the barge took about forty-five minutes, which provided a nice break from work at the beachhead. Sandy and I decided to use this time to take a tour of the settlement.

We set out to towards the second beachhead, farther down the shoreline, following the edge of the escarpment. We were careful not to trip over stone outcroppings or turn an ankle by suddenly stepping into a depression.

"Sandy, look at this! I just found it lodged in the pebbles," I called out. "What do you make of it? It looks like a tooth, maybe a whale's tooth?"

Sandy took a closer look at it. "I agree. It could be from a whale." Sandy returned the tooth, and I pocketed it as a keepsake.

On our return to the unloading site, we decided to walk farther inland, away from the escarpment. We tried to follow what we thought was a path worn in the stubbly grass. By now, darkness had made it difficult to see any hazards in the rough terrain, and as we did not have a flashlight, we kept our eye on the glow of lights at the beachhead.

All of a sudden, we discovered that we had stumbled into the dogs' sleeping area. We were surrounded by huskies, curled up on the grass asleep after their meal. We tried to be as quiet as possible, as we stepped gingerly amongst the pack. I remembered the old saying, "let sleeping dogs lie," and realized that the last thing we wanted was to be in the midst of a pack of rudely woken dogs. A few did raise their heads, sniffed the air, and barked briefly, causing us to pause in fear. We knew it would useless to try to calm them down. Not only were we strangers in their territory, but also, they would respond only to their master's tongue. We experienced several such tense moments as we continued to make our way to the beachhead and safety.

Break over, I climbed on board the barge, where my foot became stuck amongst several large sacks of flour. A young Eskimo boy saw my predicament and he helped to free me. He then proceeded to help me get off the barge. From that point on, he stuck by my side and offered to help me as best he could. We chatted back and forth, but I had difficulty understanding him even though he did have some English. I was sure he did not understand me, but this did not matter. With lots of smiles and friendly banter, we quickly became friends. As I continued working, with every opportunity my new-found friend would make a beeline towards me and shake my hand. This, accompanied by laughter and a huge grin, showed how happy he was to be my friend.

At midnight, with the knowledge that the tide was ebbing, I, along with the other seamen, returned to the ship. The Eskimo boy and I waved our goodbyes as the barge pulled away from the shoreline. Perhaps he thought I would return with the *Howe* next year, I do not know.

After the barges were hauled aboard and secured, the *Howe* weighed anchor. It was two in the morning, and Sandy and I were in our cabin fast asleep.

We arrived at the next community, Brevoort Island, two hours later. The helicopter ferried Eskimos for the medical survey, but I continued to sleep. After three hours, the medical survey was completed and the *Howe* set sail to our next destination, Frobisher Bay.

It was Saturday, September 12, and the temperature was 38°F. We saw snow flying that afternoon, but not enough to accumulate on the decks of the ship. Regardless, this was a stark reminder that winter was never very far away in the North.

Bill received a cablegram informing him that he was scheduled to fly south from Frobisher Bay in a few days. Although Bill had mentioned his intentions to leave prior to our return to Quebec City, this news jolted me. Bill and I had shared many adventures during the voyage, each one leaving an indelible mark in our memories. I was going to miss our games of cribbage, our heart-to-heart discussions, and our companionship. It was also a reminder that this shared experience was coming to an end.

At seven in the morning of September 14, I was awakened by the distinct cranking sounds of the engines in reverse; the anchor was set. We were in Frobisher Bay, at last.

# Chapter Fourteen

# Frobisher Bay, Baffin Island

Frobisher Bay[9] was a bustling hub for the Eastern Arctic, a large community with an airport and numerous buildings, including housing for those stationed in this remote region of Canada. Several people, who had been here previously, commented that I should be prepared for an eye-opening experience.

The medical survey continued as Eskimos were transported by barge to and from the quay. While I knew Frobisher Bay had a large Eskimo population, it seemed as though the number of Eskimos arriving for their medical checkups was endless. Adding to the mix were Eskimos from other communities who were disembarking so as to fly south for medical treatment not available in the North.

Regardless, the Eskimos were in high spirits, judging from the volume of their conversation and laughter, mixed with the high "EEEs" that could be heard throughout the ship. It was a joyous occasion.

There were fewer cabins to make up, as many in the medical party stayed ashore overnight; therefore, the cabin boys and a few seamen were ordered to clean all companionways. Once again, more spit and polish, as there was expectation of a visit from high-ranking government officials. Although we may have been in the homestretch, there was no time to slack off.

This was also the day Bill was set to leave the ship. I was happy for him, as he was returning home to Ottawa in order to prepare for his return to university. We spent the last few hours

---

9   Frobisher Bay was renamed Iqaluit in 1987 and became the capital of the new territory of Nunavut in 1999.

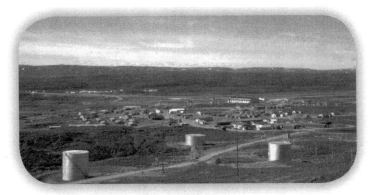

*Airport at Frobisher Bay.*
*From the Delaute family collection, courtesy of E. (Liz) Delaute Simms.*

chatting about the trip. We had shared chores, experiences, many hands of cribbage, and lots of laughter on the voyage. After supper, Bill boarded the helicopter. With Robbie Levack piloting the whirlybird, it slowly lifted off the pad at the stern of the ship, hovered briefly above the deck, then flew twice around the ship, waving goodbye. I was going to miss Bill.

The next day, guests arrived for dinner in the dining salon. When I arrived for pantry duty, I was taken aback by the sight. The tables had been set with fine, white linen tablecloths, candles, and elaborate place settings fit for royalty, in my opinion. I assumed there would be several courses for this dinner.

As I was standing near the entrance to the pantry, I caught a glimpse of the guests as they entered the dining salon. I recognized one guest, Liz Delaute. Liz and I had mutual friends, and had often seen each other at weekend dances back in Ottawa.

"How did you get to be here?" we exclaimed in unison. We chatted briefly, then Liz introduced me to her parents and sister. I could see the captain, who was standing nearby, was struggling to maintain a gracious manner for his guests. I could feel his displeasure over the fact that a lowly cabin boy was acquainted with his guests. If looks could kill, I was dead.

Liz's father, Frank Delaute, had been the assistant secretary to Governor General Vincent Massey (1952–59). In February 1959, he was appointed Administrator of the Arctic and posted to Frobisher Bay, with his wife and two daughters following a couple of months later in June.

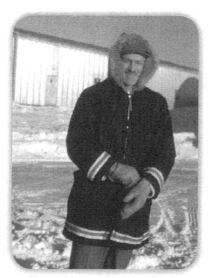

*J. Frank Delaute, Administrator of the Arctic.*
*From the Delaute family collection, courtesy of E. (Liz) Delaute Simms.*

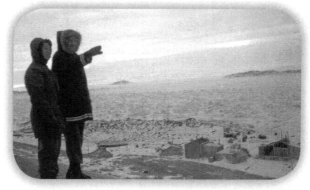

*Frank Delaute and Simione, administrative assistant and interpreter.*
*From the Delaute family collection, courtesy of E. (Liz) Delaute Simms.*

After dinner, Mr. Delaute invited Sandy Bryce and me to go ashore and visit with his family. The captain gave his permission, and we joined the Delaute family in the barge for the short trip to the quay.

We soon arrived at the Delaute home. Mr. Delaute took us on a brief tour, describing the unique features of the home. It was a long building built above ground level, containing five housing units, each a separate living space, but with only one exterior door, located in the end unit. One entered through this door, then walked through the other four units, until arriving at the Delaute unit. While this design allowed for the efficient distribution of

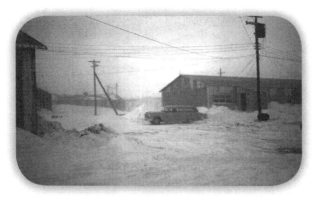

*Frobisher Bay town site.*
*From the Delaute family collection, courtesy of E. (Liz) Delaute Simms.*

heating and water, there were some obvious disadvantages in terms of privacy. Erecting the building off the ground meant that it was not subject to the pressures of permafrost and that the inhabitants were less likely to be snowed in. These buildings were the property of Northern Affairs and National Resources.

Upon completion of the short tour, we returned to the Delautes' unit, where we were shown into the living room and sat down on a comfortable sofa. It was an inviting room, and Mrs. Delaute offered refreshments of coffee and homemade cookies. What a treat after nearly three months on board ship. Over the tasty cookies, Mr. Delaute continued to tell us about many interesting and different aspects of living in the North.

At midnight, we thanked the Delautes for a delightful evening and returned to the ship. It had been a most pleasant evening, offering both an insight to the North and a wee bit of home. They were gracious hosts, and during our visit I had come to the realization that Mr. Delaute held an important position in this remote community.

We arrived at the quay on time, but there was no barge to meet us. It was a lovely moonlit night, however, with moonbeams dancing across the ripples of the bay. About forty minutes later, our solitude was broken, with the put-put of the engine as the barge splashed its way through the water, and we returned to the ship with pleasant memories of an informative, warm, and delightful visit.

Our cabin was extremely hot, stuffy, and smelly. The ducts bringing cool, fresh air from the exterior to the interior of the ship

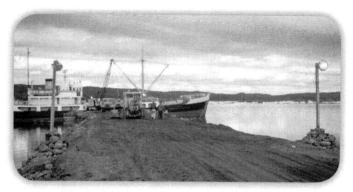

*Supply ship alongside quay at Frobisher Bay.*
*From the Delaute family collection, courtesy of E. (Liz) Delaute Simms.*

must have been clogged with soot and dust. I sought out a seaman and explained the problem. Together, we went up to clean the air filters, which were located aft of the funnel on the top deck. The ship's engines burned Bunker No. 3 oil, which not only smells bad, but also, when burned, spews out exhaust containing particles of black soot. While the seamen regularly cleaned these filters while at sea, this duty had obviously been neglected while anchored in Frobisher Bay. No wonder there was so much soot all over our beds and clothes. With the cleaning completed, cool, fresh air flowed into our cabin once again.

I finally got an opportunity to go up to the ship's Bridge (wheelhouse). This was a special treat, although I never did learn why this area was restricted. The equipment on display there, however, took my breath away, and I was impressed by the fact that I could see so much of the ship. The quartermaster, Mr. Barbeau, was at the helm (i.e., on duty), and he took pleasure in explaining the functioning of the various pieces of equipment and answering my many questions. This brief tour satisfied my curiosity, and I was now able to scratch the Bridge off my list of off-limits areas of the ship.

We sailed from Frobisher Bay in the afternoon of September 18. The sky was overcast with light snow falling. Winter was fast approaching. The rocky, treeless shoreline appeared cold and grey, relieved only by tinges of white snow nestled in the valleys.

Back home, the leaves would be turning brilliant shades of red and gold. It had been a long time since we had last seen trees.

# Chapter Fifteen

# Homeward Bound

Today, the wind blew fiercely out of the northwest. We sailed in a southerly direction across Hudson Strait towards the northeastern tip of Quebec and Labrador. It was an extremely rough sail. The ship's log recorded the wind speed as Force 7 (thirty-nine to forty-six miles per hour). According to the Beaufort scale used to classify wind speeds and its effects, this wind is described as a high wind or moderate gale. Spumes from the tops of the breaking waves were blown in streaks, an incredible sight, with wave height in these near gale conditions estimated at thirteen to nineteen feet. These were the roughest seas and highest winds I had ever experienced.

Many of those on board were feeling the effects, so they remained in their cabins. This made for a slow day to make up the cabins, but also a good test of my sea legs. I felt queasy, but no urgency to run to the lee side of the Promenade Deck and stick my head over the rail. I did go out on the windward side of the Promenade Deck, however, to see the sea literally boiling in the face of this fierce wind. The howl of the wind through the rigging and by my ears was deafening, while the spray from the waves soaked my clothing. Was it ever cold! Shivering, I sought refuge inside the warm ship; however, the fierce winds made opening and closing the heavy bulkhead doors difficult. That one brief excursion on deck was enough to satisfy my curiosity. It was a "batten down the hatches" experience, for sure.

I wondered if the officers on the Bridge were concerned about the safety of the ship in these conditions. The *Howe* was being tossed about like a cork.

Lunch was cancelled, as the constant rocking and rolling of the ship made it impossible for the galley staff to prepare and serve meals. By evening, however, the wind had abated and the sea had calmed, meaning a tasty, substantial dinner was served.

The *Howe* arrived at Port Burwell early in the morning of September 20. This small settlement was our last port of call, and one could feel the change in atmosphere as the medical staff completed this last medical survey. In short order, the seamen made preparations to raise the anchor for the last time. On the Bridge, the captain and deck officers poured over the charts, setting the course southward. We were homeward bound.

That afternoon, the medical staff hosted a cocktail party in the salon. The cabin boys were invited, as a goodwill gesture for our fine attention to detail in making up their cabins and attending to other special services throughout the journey. The chefs showed off their skills, and we enjoyed the many tasty treats served up.

Everyone was having a good time, laughing and telling stories, including the captain, who circulated among the revellers with a broad smile on his face. He would move from group to group, listening to the conversation, then adding his own comments. I attributed the captain's pleasant mood to the fact that the patrol was almost completed and he had fulfilled his mission without serious mishap. The negative feelings I perceived him having towards me surely were history.

The weather forecast for the next few days promised to be overcast with rain. Visibility from the ship was reduced; we could not even see the shoreline. We sailed into the Strait of Belle Isle, between Newfoundland and Labrador, past Point Amour on September 22. A strong following sea seemed to push the *Howe*, as eager as I was to reach our final destination. I was keen to see the historic Point Amour lighthouse, the tallest in Atlantic Canada, but, unfortunately, the weather was socked in and visibility was limited. I could not even see the beacon, let alone the separation of sea and the horizon. Disappointed, I returned to my duties. While I was unable to take pictures at the time, Fred Letto, my good friend and a native Newfoundlander, has kindly shared a few of his.

Thursday, September 24, marked the end of our thirteenth week on board the *Howe*. The past few days had been uneventful. Besides our regular duties, we were required to pass the mop in all

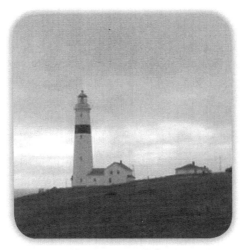

*Point Amour Lighthouse.*
*From the Letto family collection, courtesy of Fred Letto.*

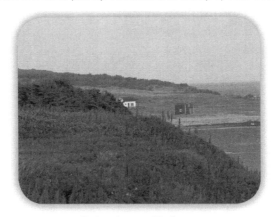

*Point Amour Harbour.*
*From the Letto family collection, courtesy of Fred Letto.*

the companionways, including stairs and walls. It was something to note how much dirt and soot had accumulated on the walls and bulkheads, settling into every nook and cranny. Other tasks included polishing the brass equipment, all under the exacting eye of Chief Steward Moreau

The seamen were kept busy bringing the Howe's exterior up to shipshape condition. They washed the bulkheads and decks, and cleaned and checked the lifeboats and fire equipment. All had to be ready for possible official visitors in Quebec City, or the Howe's next assignment.

As we passed Father Point, we picked up the river pilot and the captain's wife, who were ferried out to the ship in a motor launch. The pilot would be responsible for our course up the St. Lawrence River until we docked at the quay in Quebec City. Once again, another sign that our voyage was almost over.

Over the next few days, as we made our way up the mighty St. Lawrence, I tried to get on deck as often as possible to view the scenery. It had been some time since I had last seen trees. The weather was mainly overcast, but when the sun broke through, the view of the north shore was breathtaking. We were too far away to make out any settlements; however, the brilliance of the reds and golds along the rising shoreline made for a glorious sight.

During our last evening on board, many of the medical staff, seamen, and ship's officers were on the Promenade Deck enjoying the scenery. The *Howe* was gliding, almost noiselessly, through the waters, and everyone took great pleasure in pointing out familiar sights.

This party mood moved into the salon, where we gathered until the early morning to celebrate this last night.

Later, as I lay in bed, sleep eluded me as my thoughts skipped over a myriad scenarios that could occur the next day. I wondered if my parents, brother, and sisters would arrive in time. My father had a reputation of either not arriving or, at best, being, as he would say, properly late. An inveterate worrier, I conjured up several options for getting home to Ottawa should my parents fail to be on the quay in Quebec when we arrived.

My thoughts soon were in free fall. What changes could I expect? I had been away for a long time. Mail had come sporadically, and the letters received relayed information that was either sparse on details or sorely out of date.

Would my friends be interested in hearing of my adventures? Would my girlfriend, Liz, still be interested in me? Many had warned me that three months apart was akin to the phrase, "absence makes the heart wander." I hoped this would not be the case, but time would tell.

I also looked forward to a change in my routine. No longer would I be told what to do and when; where to go and not.

Then, there were the people. Some I would miss, others, not so much. I recalled those sage words of advice from the good Dr. Oschinsky: "This experience is character-building." Had this summer as a cabin boy really added to my character?

On these thoughts, I finally drifted off to sleep.

It seemed as though only a short while had passed when the night steward knocked on our cabin door. I would not miss these wake-up calls, either.

It was September 25. First Mate Pelletier had been right in his prediction.

Home at last!

# Afterword

**M**y tale of a memorable journey has come to an end, but this northern adventure remains a featured period in my life.

I have retained an interest in all things Northern, my attention piqued every time I hear or read something related to Canada's vast expanse beyond the tree line. During my teaching career, I would often weave recollections into lessons, taking the opportunity both to reminisce and share my love for the North.

I reiterate: it is a love, a passion, which continues to this day and which I know is shared by many who have ventured into the Land of the Midnight Sun.

During the car trip home from Quebec City on that 25th day of September, 1959, my stories kept pace with the turning of the wheels of the car as we hummed down the highway. As the bright lights of Montreal began to light up the evening horizon, I recalled our tour in search of the city's hot spots only three months before. We stopped for a steak dinner at Dinty Moore's, a popular restaurant in Montreal. I could not remember the last time I had seen steak on my menu, and I savoured every bite while relating even more adventures.

Back in the car, the last two hours flew by, punctuated with exclamations of, "Did I tell you . . ." as I launched into yet another tale.

Back at school, I found new audiences for my adventures among my friends. One little vignette would prompt a torrent of questions.

"Would you go up North again on the *Howe*?" was a question frequently asked. I had not considered this possibility. As time passed, I realized there were other interesting adventures open to me, and my experiences that summer of '59 on the *Howe* had proven that I was ready to take them on.

# Appendix A

# Interview with Liz Delaute Simms and Suzanne Delaute Allan

G iven the passage of time, I sought clarification of my diary notes during the writing of this book, including our brief visit to Frobisher Bay. I was able to contact Liz Delaute Simms hoping she could remember the *Howe*'s—and my—visit to Frobisher Bay. She and her sister, Suzanne Delaute Allan, who was twelve years old at the time, agreed to help fill in the gaps. What follows is a transcript of our conversation.

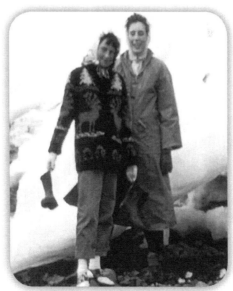

*Liz and Suzie Delaute.*
*From the Delaute family collection, courtesy of E. (Liz) Delaute Simms.*

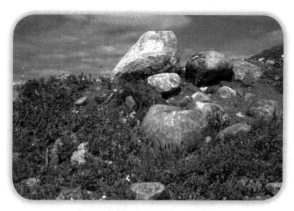

*Flowers in Frobisher Bay.*
*From the Delaute family collection, courtesy of E. (Liz) Delaute Simms.*

MA: Can you recall any memories of the dinner you and your family had on board the *Howe*?

LS: Not much, other than the excitement of being invited by the captain to dinner on THE ship. I remember being interested in getting a tour of the ship. I think the *C.D. Howe* was fairly new ... certainly the excitement of her being in port had been felt for days before you arrived.

SA: I was very impressed by the fact that the helicopter came to pick us up and take us out to the ship. We returned by boat on a beautiful starlit night, which I still remember, but I don't remember the dinner itself.

LS: Suzie and I had only been in town for a couple of months, so we had lots of new and interesting things to see and do, new people to meet. We were being included in my father's job, which was pretty special. One of the great things about living in No. 75–1 was meeting all the fascinating people coming and going, and we were learning so much at an adult level, more than we ever had at school. There were researchers of all kinds, big construction contracts of interest, the DEW Line was extending to Greenland, and operations being turned over to the Federal Electric Company, new building plans for the town site, mining engineers, weather experts, photographers, journalists, bird watchers, linguists, sociologists, medical researchers, politicians—all part of the new interest in Arctic development, many staying at the transient centre and often coming as guests for dinner at our house. The whole summer was very exciting.

SA: I remember a botanist who was studying the wild flowers. They were all very tiny by our standards, but as beautiful as any flower we knew once we appreciated their smallness. To this day, I recall this man's excitement when I see little wee wild flowers.

MA: Please describe the housing unit in which you and your family lived. Please include as much detail as possible both interior and exterior.

LS: This was a Butler Building, pre-fab steel, I think. Ours was No. 75–1.

SA: We did not live at 75–1 right away, but in a similar Butler building, where there were three apartments for NA & NR[10] staff. We moved to 75–1 in the late fall of 1959.

LS: One end of the unit was a private apartment for the Administrator of the Arctic, in which there were three bedrooms, bathroom, living room, kitchen, pantry, dining room, and a private entrance at the front. There was a door at the back end of our apartment that led into the "transient quarters," a long hallway with rooms off it, probably a bathroom there, too. I'm not sure how many rooms or suites, but they were used for people on their way to or from the smaller communities, sometimes for medical appointments; sometimes the residents were researchers or VIPs on government business. There was a back entrance to the outside from the transient quarters' end of the building; we did have privacy at our end because we had our own front door.

Our apartment was nice inside, all standard government-issue furniture: solid maple, colonial style, comfortable. We may have had a few personal items that my mum had brought from Ottawa, but not much. She made it feel homey, though.

MA: How accurate is my description of the utilities? If you recall details, please expand. Who paid for these services?

LS: The toilets were serviced by the honey wagon, an orange truck which did the rounds daily and took away the sewage. In some of the units, the honey buckets were emptied manually by an employed person who came in daily and carried the toilet buckets from the bathrooms to the honey wagon, then cleaned and returned them to the bathrooms. In our unit, because of the transient centre, I think there might have been a hose system out to the truck.

---

10 Northern Affairs and National Resources.

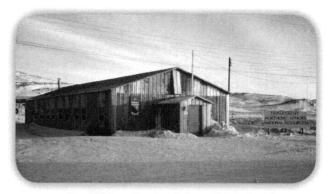

*Butler Building, home of the Delaute family.*
*From the Delaute family collection, courtesy of E. (Liz) Delaute Simms.*

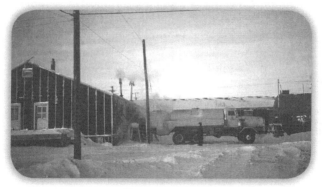

*Honey wagon.*
*From the Delaute family collection, courtesy of E. (Liz) Delaute Simms.*

SA: I remember Mum and me visiting someone in Apex Hill[11] once and the honey wagon worker arrived and grinned a very toothless grin as he carried the bucket from the bathroom out through the living room where we were visiting and out to the honey wagon.

LS: When we lived in 75–1, there must have been a utility room down the hall—furnace room, electrical boxes, and water storage tanks. The water for the house came by truck, daily, and a hose system was used to fill a tank that was in a utility room, which would have been heated, inside the building. Deliveries could be erratic in really cold weather.

---

11 Apex (Inuktitut Niaqunngut) is a small community near Frobisher Bay (Iqaluit). Historically, Apex was where most Inuit lived when Iqaluit was a military site and off-limits to anyone not working at the base.

My recollection of Frobisher in 1959 does not include buildings on stilts, nor do I remember a utility corridor pipeline.

SA: I think the Apex houses were on stilts.

LS: I think this type of structure was used in Tuktoyaktuk, Inuvik, and the Western Arctic.

I don't know how my parents paid for the apartment, or the services. When I worked for NANR in Povungnituk, Quebec, in 1962, my housemate and I paid a monthly fee, which was deducted from our salary. This included rent for our house and a year's supply of food. I suspect this is how my parents paid for the accommodation in No. 75-1. When my husband and I lived in Lake Harbour[12] in 1964–66 [working for the Hudson's Bay Company], we paid $100 a month for our furnished, four-bedroom house and a year's supply of food. This amount was deducted from George's paycheque. We didn't use cash while we lived there. Everything was recorded on our accounts in the Winnipeg head office, and if we needed something, we just recorded it on the store accounts: gas, skidoo, fabric, extras. Again, the house was furnished comfortably—all services were included.

MA: Your family needed supplies [food, drink, etc.]; can you recall how this problem was solved?

LS: My father left Ottawa for Frobisher in February 1959. My mother completed the sale of our house on Rideau Terrace [Ottawa] then she, my youngest sister, Suzie, and I joined him in June of that year. We were settled in Frobisher at the beginning of July. In February of '59, my mother would have submitted her order for groceries and supplies to the NANR office in Ottawa, having figured out what she thought we would need for the following year. The staff at head office had excellent inventory lists that she would have used to make her order; also she had been quartermaster at Guide camp, so had a pretty good idea of where to start. The complete order would have arrived on one of the ships that came in during the summer and were unloaded at the beach at Apex Hill. There, all the incoming shipments were sorted, identified, and delivered to the Bay, government stores, or the individual houses. We unpacked and stored our stores order in a storage room in the

---

12 Kimmirut, Nunavut.

house and tried not to eat all the good stuff first!

SA: Because we were to move to 75–1 in the fall and our year's supply of groceries had arrived in late August, everything remained in boxes in our kitchen. In mid-September, my mother had gone to B.C. for our sister Val's wedding. I kept noticing a strong smell of Javex and finally saw liquid at the bottom of one of the boxes. Dad and I did some unpacking and found a Javex bottle packed on its side. The Javex had eaten through the metal cap. I don't recall it damaging anything else!

LS: My father would also have made a liquor order for the year before he left in February. In my case, when I went to Povungnituk in '62, my housemate and I neglected to think about this aspect of our creature comforts, and subsequently made good friends of the Austin Airways pilots, who would do our liquor shopping in Timmins and bring our supplies in by air; a more costly approach! I remember later on, some of the families found a food supplier in Montreal who would send group orders in on Nordair, which had fairly regular, scheduled flights by then on a DC-4.

MA: Any recollections of the white-sided buildings with the red roofs situated along the embankment just up from the beachhead?

LS: These would be the Hudson's Bay Company buildings in Apex Hill. Frobisher Bay, in 1959, consisted of several subdivisions. The Strategic Air Command[13]complex was high up on the hill above the airport. The airport was at the centre of the Department of Transport section. The main "town" of Frobisher Bay was all of the Transport holdings around the airport, including their staff accommodations, and their own supply wharves. The administrative area adjacent to the DOT[14] lands was where we lived; the department heads lived in Butler Buildings around the main Admin Building—No. 79. Both the DOT and the NANR Admin section together were called the town site; the RCMP headquarters, the Anglican church, the school, and the hospital were also here. Nearby was a shantytown of thrown together buildings where a lot of the native Eskimos lived. It had an Inuit

13 USAF-SAC
14 Department of Transport

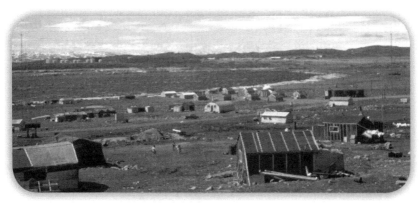

*Shantytown 1.*
*From the Delaute family collection, courtesy of E. (Liz) Delaute Simms.*

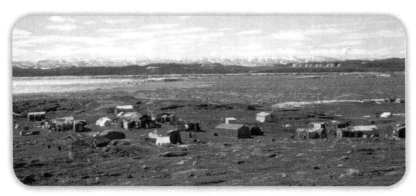

*Shantytown 2.*
*From the Delaute family collection, courtesy of E. (Liz) Delaute Simms.*

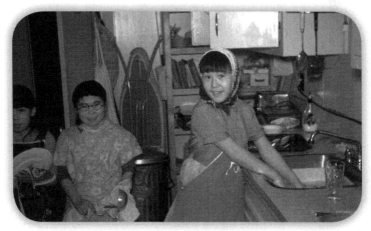

*Mother's happy helpers.*
*From the Delaute family collection, courtesy of E. (Liz) Delaute Simms.*

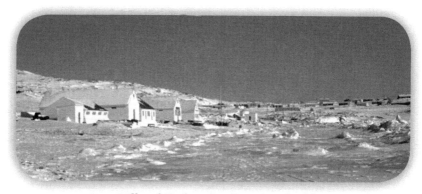

*Apex Hill and Hudson Bay Company buildings.*
*From the Delaute family collection, courtesy of E. (Liz) Delaute Simms.*

name, which I can't remember, maybe Iqaluit?

SA: Yes, I think the shantytown was called Iqaluit. I remember seeing a house that had been built using scrap lumber, some of which was from the packing cases that our few personal belongings had been shipped up in. "J.F. Delaute" was stamped on the outside of the packing cases, which were subsequently used on the little house.

LS: About five miles east of this area was Apex Hill. Most of the government employees lived in government houses in Apex. These were not Butler Buildings. They were older, probably wooden, pre-fab types. The Hudson's Bay Company had a lot of land, the main store, and warehouse buildings in Apex, all managed by Newfoundlander Gordon Rennie. Apex is where all the HBC and NANR supplies—other than DOT—were unloaded; this is where we did our "shopping"—not that we needed much—and where a

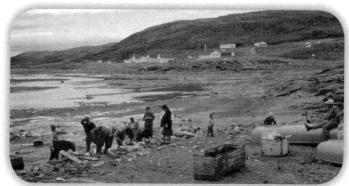

*Food preparation after a hunt.*
*From the Delaute family collection, courtesy of E. (Liz) Delaute Simms.*

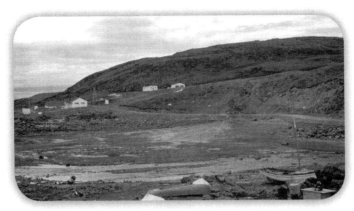

*Tide out.*
*From the Delaute family collection, courtesy of E. (Liz) Delaute Simms.*

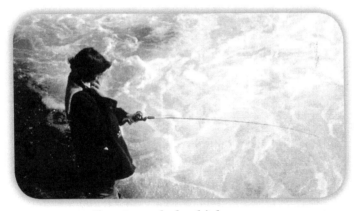

*Shopping at the local fishmongers.*
*From the Delaute family collection, courtesy of E. (Liz) Delaute Simms.*

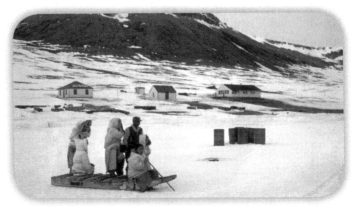

*Family on a komatik (sled).*
*From the Delaute family collection, courtesy of E. (Liz) Delaute Simms.*

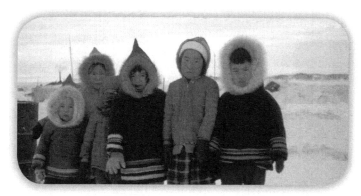

*Children on their way to school.*
*From the Delaute family collection, courtesy of E. (Liz) Delaute Simms.*

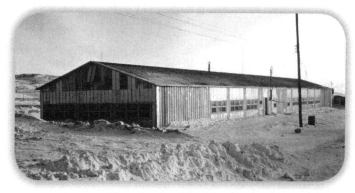

*The school at Frobisher Bay.*
*From the Delaute family collection, courtesy of E. (Liz) Delaute Simms.*

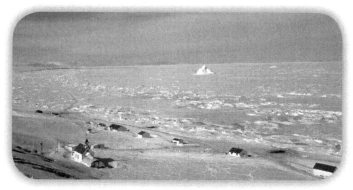

*The Anglican church, Frobisher Bay.*
*From the Delaute family collection, courtesy of E. (Liz) Delaute Simms.*

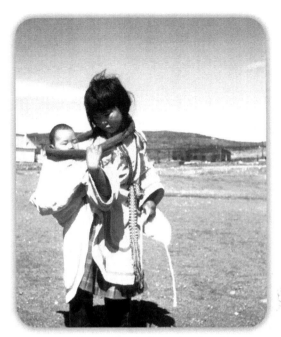

*Mother with a baby in her hood.*
*From the Delaute family collection, courtesy of E. (Liz) Delaute Simms.*

lot of the social events took place for the government employees and their families.

SA: I seem to remember that everyone was attempting to shop for toilet paper in the few months before the ships came in with the upcoming year's order. Those who had ordered using the department's suggested quantities of certain essentials were trying to trade their excess of ketchup for toilet paper. I think Mum had figured out the correct amounts before placing her order.

LS: There was an old school bus used for public transportation back and forth between the town site and Apex. I remember Charlie was the driver.

SA: Charlie's wife sometimes rode the bus halfway to Apex and got off. One day, Mum asked Charlie why she got off, and he replied, "To hunt for their food."

Appendix B

# The Eastern Arctic Patrol

"Times have changed in Canada's Eastern Arctic. Communities which once knew splendid isolation of another world are now in almost daily communication with the cities to the south. Aircraft and radio have made neighbours of distant places and even across the lonely ice-strewn water passes a growing traffic of ships. The changes in the Eastern Arctic Patrol over the decades have mirrored the changes in Canada's Eastern Arctic. Its development is a reflection of the opening of Canada's distant northern territory."[15]

Several voyages were made to the Eastern Arctic in the early years of the twentieth century. Initial expeditions were undertaken by the well-known and Arctic-experienced Captain J.E. Bernier. "In 1944, a vigorous campaign was started to control the worst plague of the Arctic, tuberculosis, and on the last complete patrol by the *Nascopie* there were no less than six medical officers, an X-ray technician, a dentist, an oculist and optical technician, and two nurses. In 1947, the *Nascopie* sank on a reef off Cape Dorset. "In 1944, a vigorous campaign was started to control the worst plague of the Arctic, tuberculosis, and on the last complete patrol by the *Nascopie* there were no less than six medical officers, an X-Ray technician, a dentist, an oculist and optical technician, and two nurses. By 1950 the *C.D. Howe*, the first ship built as an Arctic

15 R.A.J. Phillips, "The Eastern Arctic Patrol," *Canadian Geographical Journal*, Vol. 14, No. 5 (May 1957), p. 191.

Patrol vessel, came into service and a new era began to dawn."[16]

The *C.D. Howe*, named after a prominent federal cabinet minister in the governments of William Lyon Mackenzie King and Louis St. Laurent, was built by the Davie Shipbuilding Company, of Lauzon, Quebec. She was equipped with the latest navigational equipment, plus a helicopter for ice reconnaissance and transportation of personnel. The ship was strengthened for limited icebreaking.

The ship was mandated to bring medical services and supplies to the numerous Eskimo settlements in the Eastern Arctic. The up-to-date medical facilities on board included surgical theatres, an X-ray suite, sick bays, and dental facilities.

The *C.D. Howe* had a crew of approximately fifty-eight and medical and support staff of approximately fifty-eight, as well. There was accommodation for up to thirty Eskimos, who were either travelling south for treatment for tuberculosis or returning home.

Many Eskimos were evacuated during this time to southern sanatoriums for an extended period of treatment and recuperation. At the conclusion of successful treatment, they returned to their settlements, rejoining their families as passengers on board the *Howe*. The incidence of tuberculosis declined around the same time as a hospital was opened in Frobisher Bay in 1964.

The *Howe*, however, continued service in the Eastern Arctic, albeit with significant changes to its mandate. Eventually, the matter of the relevance of the services became an issue among government departments, and it became difficult to acquire medical personnel for an extended period of floating isolation. In 1968, the decision was made to end the patrol that season.

Little information exists on the *C.D. Howe*; however, upon request, a friend doing research at the Maritime Museum in Vancouver took a look at the *C.D. Howe* file. There it was discovered that the *Howe* was sold to Vestgron Mines of Vancouver around 1970; in 1971, she was sent to Greenland to be used as a floating base camp for mining exploration.

16 Ibid., p. 193

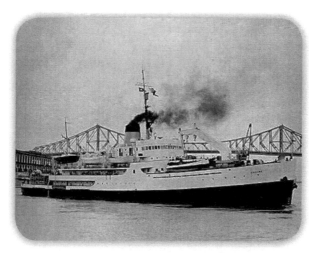

*C.D. Howe, Port of Montreal. Unknown.*

### CGS *C.D. Howe* 1950–70

| | |
|---|---|
| Builder: | Davie Shipbuilding Ltd., Lauzon, Quebec |
| Date Completed: | 1950 |
| Tonnage: | 3628 (gross) |
| Dimensions: | 295 x 50 x 19.5 (ft); 91 x 15.4 x 6 (m) |
| Machinery: | Twin-screw steam uniflow, 4000 IHP |
| Speed: | 13.5 kts |

A unique, ice-strengthened Northern Service vessel named for former minister of transport and wartime minister of munitions and supplies, the *C.D. Howe* was employed on the Eastern Arctic Patrol and performed exemplary service in the North for twenty years, assisting shipping in the Gulf of St. Lawrence during the winter. In her last years, she also acted as a training vessel for Coast Guard College cadets. She was sold in 1970 and converted to an accommodation ship for workers at the Black Angel mine in Maarmorilik Fjord, Greenland.

From 1950 to 1970, the *C.D. Howe* made annual voyages to northern Labrador and the south and east coasts of Baffin Island, stopping at every coastal settlement and station, and also at points on Ellesmere Island. There was accommodation for eighty-eight passengers and fifty-eight crew. She carried Department of Northern Affairs, National Resources employees and RCMP members.

The provision of medical and dental services was probably her most important role. She had a well-equipped hospital (operating rooms, X-ray facilities, ancillary medical support, and complete dental suite), while medical officers included two doctors, two nurses, and one or two dentists. She was the first Department of Transport ship to carry a helicopter.[17]

In 1953, the *C.D. Howe* carried Inuit families, with their sled dogs, kayaks, and other possessions, from Port Harrison[18] on the eastern side of Hudson Bay, to Craig Harbour on Ellesmere Island, later moved to Grise Fiord, which had easier access for supply vessels. The objective was to provide new hunting grounds and to populate some of the more northerly locations in the archipelago.

17 Charles D. Maginley and Bernard Collin, *The Ships of Canada's Marine* Services (St. Catharines, Ontario: Vanwell Publishing Ltd., 2004), p.p 145–46.
18 Inukjuak, Quebec.

# Appendix C

# Statistical Information

**SS C.D. Howe:**
Eastern Arctic Patrol Ship
Designed by Milne, Gilmore & German, naval architects,
 Montreal, for the Department of Transport.
Built by Davie Shipbuilding and Repair Co. Ltd., Lauzon, Quebec,
 1949.
Christened and launched September 7, 1949.
Sponsor: Mrs. W.H. Howe.

**Principal Dimensions:**
Length overall: 295 ft
Breadth: 50 ft
Draught: 18 ft. 6 in.
Tonnage: 3,628 tons
Machinery: steam uniflow
Engines: 2 x 2000 IHP (4000 IHP)
Boilers: 2
Propellers: 4 blades 10.5 ft. dia.
Speed (loaded): 13.5 knots
Radius of action: 10,000 miles
Crew: 58
Passengers: 88 (58 medical, 30 Eskimo)

**Classification:** Lloyd's Register of Shipping—Highest class for a vessel for "foreign voyages," "with free board," "metallic arc welded," and "strengthened for navigation in ice."

Outfitted with the latest communications and navigation equipment. Additional equipment for hydrographers' use included.

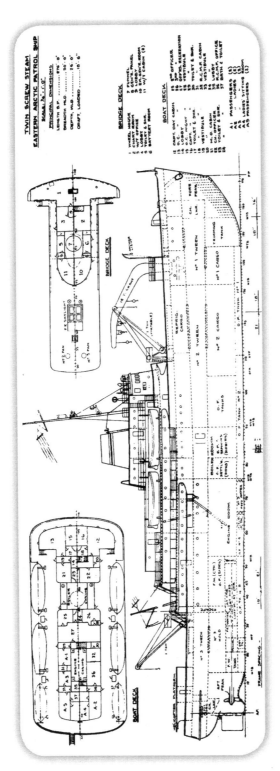

*Schematic of C.D. Howe.*
*Department of Transport.*

Other onboard equipment: cargo cranes, buoy crane (15-ton goose neck), life-saving equipment with sufficient capacity for the crew and passengers.

Helicopter platform located aft. Helicopter on board as per current practices governing operation in northern waters. The helicopter was used mainly for ice reconnaissance and emergency transportation. Personnel included the helicopter pilot and the mechanic.

**Description:** raked stem and cruiser stern, two continuous decks and three cargo holds.

**Main Deck:** steering gear compartment, laundries for passengers and crew, rest rooms and cabins for the crew.

**Upper Deck:** quarters for engineer officers, stewards, and Eskimos; carpenter shop, stores, cold cargo and stores, bakery, galley, and scullery; and mess rooms for officers, stewards, oilers, firemen, and seamen; hospital unit, including a well-equipped sick bay with berths for six persons, an operating room, an X-ray room with adjacent darkroom, a dispensary, and adequate washroom facilities. Patient needs attended to by a medical officer, dentist, and sick bay attendant.

**Promenade Deck:** twenty double cabins, dining salon (passengers, captain, and ranking officers), and lounge.

**Boat Deck:** accommodation for the captain and officer commanding the Eastern Arctic Patrol (OCEAP). Each has a suite comprising day and night cabins and washroom. In addition, four double passenger cabins, two of which are reserved for ladies, ensuite with sitting room and toilet facilities, an RCMP suite with a large office, and an officers' recreation room.

**Bridge Deck:** wheelhouse, chart room, wireless/telegrapher office and cabin, emergency generator, and battery room.[19]

---

19 "SS *C.D. Howe*," Eastern Arctic patrol ship. Designed by Milne, Gilmour & German, Naval Architects Montreal for the Department of Transport. Built by Davie Shipbuilding and Repairing Co. Ltd., Lauzon, Quebec, 1949. (LAC 629.gmfu CIII) [Montreal? : s.n.], 1949. — 20 leaves : ill. ; 22 cm. — AMICUS No. 4104013.

# Appendix D

# Manifest 1959 (unofficial)

**Ship's Officers:**
Captain/Master: J.M. Desrosiers
First Mate: Pelletier
Second Mate:
Third Mate / Purser: A. Brie
W/T Chief: Laxton
Officer-in-Charge EAP: Dr. A.H. Stevens, MD
Helicopter Pilot: Robbie Levack
Helicopter Engineer: Dick Preston
Quartermaster: Barbeau
Postmaster:
Carpenter:
Night Steward: Jacques Jolicoeur (Joli-Coeur)
Chief Steward: Moreau
First Steward: Louis
Second Steward: Armand

Cabin Boys (English): Murray Ault, Robert (Bob) Ferguson, William (Bill) Kendall, and Alexander (Sandy) Bryce.
Cabin Boys (French): There were four lads in this group.
Seamen: Jean-Marc Thibideau

**Engineering Staff**
Chief Engineer:
Second Engineer:

**Staff:**

*Medical Staff:*

Dr. A.H. Stevens, Eastern Region Office, Officer Commanding
    Eastern Arctic Patrol

Dr. Ruth McLeese, Eastern Region Office Medical Officer

Dr. R.M. Lane, radiologist (first half), Victoria, British Columbia

Dr. R.L. Empey, radiologist (second half), Mountain Sanatorium,
    Hamilton, Ontario

Dr. Roy Smithurst, dental officer, Vancouver, British Columbia

Miss Yvonne Desrochers, PHN, INHS, nurse

Miss Faith Gange, RN, Mountain Sanatorium, Hamilton, Ontario

Mr. Norman Harper, X-ray technician, Eastern Region Office

Mr. Cort Beckingham, technician's assistant (student), Ottawa,
    Ontario

Miss Jane Weetaltuk, INHS, ward aide and interpreter, Moose
    Factory, Ontario

Miss Lizzie Kauki, interpreter and registrar, Payne Bay,[20] Quebec

Miss Elsie Styres, INHS, secretary (second half) Ohsweken,
    Ontario

*Additional Nursing Staff*: Madeline Onslow and Kay Denneny

*Anthropologist*: Dr. L. Oschinsky, physical anthropologist,
    Victoria Museum, Ottawa, Ontario

*Interpreter*: Alex

**Hydrographic Survey Team:**

Two motorized craft for inshore work and related hydrographic
duties, the *Greb* and the *Shag*. There was a special cabin on the
Main Deck containing hydrographic equipment and recording
devices, which were in continuous operation.

*Greb:*

Captain: Mr. R. Meredith

Cox: R. Maranda

Gas Engineer: J.B. Metayer

Seaman: Dave Simpson

---

20 Kangirsuk, Quebec.

*Shag:*
Captain: Mr. W. Henry
Cox: F. Lepine
Gas Engineer: J. Monroe
Seaman: A. Vigeant

**Eastern Arctic Patrol 1959 Travel Statistics:**
Total Hours steamed:1,338.02 hours
Mileage covered during trip:11,689 miles
Average speed:8.74 knots

*Author's Note: This manifest was prepared from the author's personal diary and documents obtained from the Library and Archives Canada. Its accuracy is limited to the noted references.*

# Bibliography

## Articles

Cavell, Janice, and Jeff Noakes. "The Origins of Canada's First Eastern Arctic Patrol, 1919–22." *Polar Record*, Vol. 45, No. 233 (2001).

Grant, Shelagh D. "A Case of Compounded Error: The Inuit Resettlement Project, 1953, and the Government Response, 1990." *Northern Perspectives*, Vol. 19, No. 1 (Spring 1991).

Mackinnon, C.S. "Canada's Eastern Arctic Patrol 1922–68." *Polar Record*, Vol. 27, No. 161 (1991).

Phillips, R.A.J. "The Eastern Arctic Patrol." *Canadian Geographical Journal*, Vol. 14, No. 5 (May 1957).

## Books

Copland, Dudley. *Livingstone of the Arctic*. Lancaster, Ontario: Canadian Century Publishers, Second Printing, 1978.

Maginley, Charles Douglas, and Bernard Collin. *The Ships of Canada's Marine Services*. St. Catharines, Ontario: Vanwell Publishing Ltd., 2004.

Pratt, E.J. *Collected Poems of E.J. Pratt*. 2nd ed. Toronto, Ontario: Macmillan Company of Canada Ltd., 1958.

Service, Robert W. *Collected Poems of Robert Service*. Toronto, Ontario: McGraw-Hill Ryerson, 1960.

## Government[21]

37th annual Eastern Arctic Patrol—Ottawa: Department of Northern Affairs and National Resources, Editorial and Information Division, 1958. —4p. ; 28 cm.—AMICUS No. 22430952.

Annual Report 1960–1961. Department of Transport, Ottawa, Canada.

Annual Report 1959–1960. Department of Transport, Ottawa, Canada (reference to the *C.D. Howe*, *N.B. McLean*, *d'Iberville*, SS *Federal*

---

21 There are brief reports of the Eastern Arctic Patrol in the annual reports for the department that administered Northern affairs. As responsibility for Northern affairs shifted from department to department, the reports dealing with the patrol appear in different departmental annual reports, depending on the time period. For 1959–60, the patrol was under the administration of the Department of Northern Affairs and National Resources.

*Voyager,* and MV *Irvingwood,* p. 27–28).

Annual Report 1958–1959. Department of Transport, Ottawa, Canada.

Canada. Department of Northern Affairs and National Resources. Annual Report—[Ottawa : Queen's Printer, 1954–1966]—v. : ill., fold. col. maps.—ISSN 0576-1387—AMICUS No. 1576083.

Canada. Department of Northern Affairs and National Resources. Eastern Arctic Patrol—1957—15 p.—AMICUS No. 29124261.

"SS *C.D. Howe.*" Eastern Arctic patrol ship / designed by Milne, Gilmore & German for the Department of Transport; built by Davie Shipbuilding and Repairing Co.—[Montreal? : s.n.], 1949.—20 leaves: ill. ; 22 cm.— AMICUS No. 4104013.

# About the Author

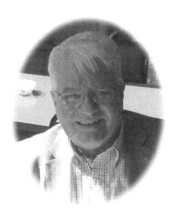

Photo by Judie Ault.

Murray Ault was born, raised, and educated in Ottawa, Ontario, where he taught history and economics for more than thirty years. He holds degrees from Carleton University and the University of Waterloo.

After retiring from the Ottawa Board of Education in 1996, he accepted an invitation by Statistics Canada to develop and write a case study for publication on their education website, utilizing the data program, ESTAT: *An Analysis of a Colonial Industry: Shipbuilding in Nova Scotia, 1861*. He also assisted in the administration of "The Teachers' Institute on Canadian Parliamentary Democracy," a program sponsored by the Speakers of the House of Commons and Senate and the Parliamentary Library.

His interest in the Canadian North has continued unabated since that summer of 1959 when he served as cabin steward aboard the *C.D. Howe*.